HIATAL HERNIA SYNDROME:

The Mother of All Illness?

Guide to Self-Healing

Theodore A. Baroody, N.D., D.C., Ph.D., C.N.C.

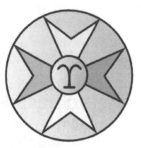

HOLOGRAPHIC HEALTH PRESS
119 Pigeon St.
Waynesville, NC 28786-4357
Website: www.holographichealth.com

DISCLAIMER

The information in this book is given strictly for educational and research purposes. The author and publisher do not prescribe or recommend, nor assume any responsibility. In no way should this information be considered a substitute for competent health care by the professional of your choice. In the event you use this information without your doctor's approval, you are prescribing for yourself, which is your constitutional right.

For information and ordering write:
HOLOGRAPHIC HEALTH, INC.
119 Pigeon St. Waynesville, NC 28786
1-800-566-1522
Website: www.holographichealth.com
ISBN: 0-9619595-2-5

DEDICATION

This book is lovingly dedicated
to the worldwide millions
suffering from this syndrome.
May it bring them comfort.

Table of Contents

i

DIAGRAMS

PHOTOS

PREFACE

I have been writing, researching and alleviating the diverse symptoms produced by this dangerous condition in literally thousands of people for over 20 years. After this length of time and amount of experience, it is obvious that the H.H.S. is much more than merely the "insidious link to major illness," as I first named it. **It is the mother of all illness.** Every chronic condition (excluding sudden traumas like auto accidents, falls, wounds, etc) is the *direct* result of some aspect of digestive dysfunction. The H.H.S. does not lead to more problems; it is the mother that births these problems. Time makes the imbalances grow and damage the rest of the body systems. It still baffles me that this deadly syndrome is taken so lightly by allopathic and alternative practitioners alike. The idea that some drug or food supplement can correct this problem quickly is ludicrous. This problem takes time and consistency to be addressed properly. Few dangerous physical maladies go away quickly, and take time. The H.H.S. is dangerous; make no mistake about that.

What is even more dangerous are the constant imbalances brought about by the HHS. These lead to any and all maladies known to mankind. The particular illness developed is unique to his/her physiology and genetic makeup. Have no illusions; the more serious imbalances could manifest in time, depending upon the two previously mentioned factors.

My files are replete with people from coast to coast and abroad whose pain has been alleviated. Amazing stories by those employing these techniques continue to pour in daily. They report multiple success rates with symptoms ranging from leukemia to leg cramps and everything in-between. I have seen cases improve, stemming from mild paralysis to projectile vomiting. I am awed and humbled at the testimonials from our suffering public and the manner in which this simple set of harmless maneuvers for the HHS brought them relief.

There is no doubt after many years of wrestling with this invisible plague that my original statistics of 85% of our population being afflicted with the Hiatal Hernia Syndrome to a greater or lesser extent are accurate - maybe even low. **Digestion is the key. Without the digestive system completely "on line", all other systems are doomed to break down eventually.**
Vagus nerve disruption by the Hiatal Hernia Syndrome is the

major cause. Dr. Carey Reams, probably the most eminent biochemist of our time, stated again and again that illness begins with vagus nerve problems. The vagus nerve, extensively explored in this book, is the portal of entry for illness in the body. The Hiatal Hernia Syndrome pinches and therefore causes this dangerous instability.

What can you do? Following the guidelines in this book can help tremendously. Since the recommendations are harmless, one has nothing to lose by attempting same for at least six weeks. If no results are obtained, then the client and practitioner will want to look deeper. Recent surgical advances for hiatal hernia repair are a little less risky than they were when I started writing about this syndrome over twenty years ago. Yet, I have still seen scant evidence that surgery is the answer except in extreme cases.

These are not the situations that are addressed in this book. Many doctors, after extensive exams, will tell us that most people have a small hiatal hernia, but that it is no problem and the client can live with it. Surgery is not recommended to these victims as a general rule, and the problem is brushed aside with some type of palliative drug.

I have endeavored to confirm clinically every word regarding the dangers of this syndrome. I remain steadfast in my views on this subject; because I have seen thousands live more productive, satisfying lives as a result of this work. It is toward a healthy future for those remaining millions of HHS sufferers that I am bound by God to preserve these teachings until all are aware of them.

Dr. Theodore A. Baroody 2007

INTRODUCTION

A cyclone is spinning -- an insidious gale of indeterminable magnitude. It affects all races, latitudes and longitudes. It strikes young and old alike. It masquerades as most of the illnesses from which we suffer. It is devastating world health, leaving us silently crippled.

Overlooked for centuries, it now takes special toll in times of high stress living. It revels in discord, misunderstood physiology and poor diet.

I call it a syndrome. Only a syndrome could slip its guileful hand underneath the attention of all manner of health providers and create such subtle havoc. Only a syndrome could catapult the planet into massive infirmities of one type or another. Only a syndrome could act as the underlying cause for such pandemic problems.

This is a book for you -- the bewildered, the discouraged, the one who is not altogether well, who wants to know why, who asks and is not told.

It is for you who suffer symptomatic aches and pains that occur seemingly without rhyme or reason. It is for you the chronic stomach sufferer, with continuous or intermittent gastric distress.

It is for the victim of an entire gamut of debilitating illnesses which are linked at base core, yet are usually diagnosed and treated ineffectively as separate problems. The real disorder is not readily evident as the controlling factor of such seemingly unrelated conditions as heart, kidney, gall bladder malfunctions, and others.

Why are the drugs for temporary relief of such distresses the number one sellers today? Why are the public's increasing clamors for reliable information and help appearing now in all kinds periodicals, practically ignored? Even when an authority responds, it is most often with traditional jargon leaving you, the patient, more confused and frustrated than before.

Do you wonder why you frequently bloat, belch excessively, why you can't breathe deeply anymore? Even as you read, do you wonder why you always feel tired, or underfed (no matter what you eat), why you are unexplainably anxious at times? Is your arsenal of aluminum derivative palliative medications close by so you can gulp them down hoping for some relief?

Over the years, I have used many names to describe this

syndrome. You will see it referenced throughout the book by such names as: the mother of all illness, the insidious link to major illness, the great trickster, and the great masquerader. All of these are good descriptions but none of them adequately explain the health horror that I watch this syndrome reek upon the population.

In this book you will discover factual reports, and simple, effective therapies for dealing with this major lurking basis of encompassing illness.

I call it the "**HIATAL HERNIA SYNDROME**".

Chapter 1

HIATAL HERNIA SYNDROME - WHAT DOES IT MEAN?

The **hiatus** is the special hole in the diaphragm, the breathing muscle, through which the esophagus normally passes to become the stomach. **Hernia** is the term for a weakened - in this case, stretched or torn muscle. If for any reason, the diaphragmatic muscle is weakened or torn, the stomach will be forced upward through the diaphragm, creating this problematical condition.

The tricky thing is that the stomach does not have to protrude far into the diaphragm to cause all kinds of bewildering symptoms. Yet, more deceptive is the fact that many times it moves up for only a few minutes or a few hours, and then drops back into place leaving the victim more confused than ever. That is why I call the HHS by so many names. In this case, the HHS is "the great trickster."

The stomach can also simply shove up against the diaphragm without tearing or penetrating it. This can cause the same problems as if it actually had torn the diaphragm. In this scenario, I call the HHS "the great masquerader". Imbalances occur from this type of involvement because the stomach pinches and disrupts the function of the vagus nerve as it enters into that area and interferes with the movement of the diaphragm muscle by not letting it move up and down during the breathing cycle. This is the situation which we see a great deal of the time. That is why I refer to it mostly as a syndrome. I do not do any x-rays or CAT scans or MRIs to confirm the HHS. If I am suspicious of the presence of a hiatal hernia and the patient needs more convincing, I send them for further tests. Otherwise, I go by the symptoms displayed and see if the correction will stop the symptoms, which it does ninety-five percent of the time. If realignment of the stomach does not stop or slow down the symptoms, then I know I am probably not dealing with HHS disruption. I am primarily interested in the disruption the stomach causes as it pinches the vagus nerve.

This diaphragmatic interference, without actually tearing the muscle and being diagnosed technically as a hiatal hernia, can still be just as painful and disruptive to the entire body systems as an actual tear in the diaphragmatic muscle.

The rebalancing of this problem can be accomplished by using the techniques given in this book. This will give one time to control the hernia until the "syndrome" has fully healed. In other words, the muscle (diaphragm) must have time to mend the hole (hiatus) so the stomach won't jump up and start causing these multi-faceted problems all over again.

Unless one has a medical diagnosis and x-rays to prove the tear is healed, one may never know for sure. What this author is offering is not a way to heal this tear conclusively, although that is the goal. What I am hoping is to give the client as much relief from this syndrome as possible, while allowing the body as much time as it needs to either mend the diaphragm or reposition the stomach so that the client will not have vagus nerve disruption or other gastrointestinal distresses associated with this imbalance.

When the HHS situation occurs in which body systems directly outside of the gastrointestinal system are involved, I call the HHS "the insidious link". This is because the HHS creates the groundwork for other major illnesses in the body.

You are only as well as your stomach's ability to:
1. Stay in its proper place
2. Digest food properly
3. Assimilate food properly
4. Distribute nutrients from the food properly
5. Eliminate waste from the bowels properly

Chapter 2

MULTI-FACETED SYMPTOMS OF THE HIATAL HERNIA SYNDROME

I have come to discount almost nothing that the HHS cannot produce in the form of discomfort. The fragile nature of the entire digestive system can be upset so easily by so many different factors, which lead to the many ills that prevail.

HIATAL HERNIA CHECKLIST

Review the checklist. If you find symptoms that apply, you may suspect vagus nerve interference and possible hiatal hernia involvement. When either of these is present, the correct ratio of alkaline to acid will be altered and create acid wastes leading to ill health.

DIGESTIVE DIFFICULTIES

1) ___ Belching
2) ___ Bloating
3) ___ Sensitivity at the waist
4) ___ Intestinal gas
5) ___ Regurgitation
6) ___ Hiccups
7) ___ Lack or limitation of appetite
8) ___ Nausea
9) ___ Vomiting
10) ___ Diarrhea
11) ___ Constipation
12) ___ Colic in children

BREATHING AND CIRCULATION PROBLEMS

1) ___ Deep breathing curtailed
2) ___ Overall fatigue and exhaustion
3) ___ Tendency to swallow air
4) ___ Allergies
5) ___ Dry tickling cough
6) ___ Full feeling at the base of throat
7) ___ Pain or burning in upper chest
8) ___ Pressure in the chest

Hiatal Hernia Syndrome

9) ___Pain in the left side of chest
10) ___Heartburn
11) ___Pressure below breastbone

12) ___ Lung pain
13) ___ Rapid heartbeat
14) ___ Rapid rise in blood pressure

STRUCTURAL COMPLAINTS

1) ___Left shoulder pain, pain in left arm, pain in left side of neck
2) ___Right shoulder pain
3) ___Pain between the shoulder blades
4) ___Joint pain in extremities

5) ___ TMJ - Temporo-Mandibular Joint pain
6) ___ Bruxism - Grinding teeth in sleep
7) ___ Localized or overall spinal pain
8) ___ Headaches

STRESS

1) ___Dizziness
2) ___Shakiness
3) ___Mental Confusion
4) ___Anxiety attacks

5) ___Insomnia
6) ___ Hyperactivity in children

OTHER AILMENTS

1) ___Craving for sugar or alcohol
2) ___Candida Albicans
3) ___Menstrual or prostate problems

4) ___ Urinary difficulties
5) ___ Hoarseness
6) ___ Obesity

The following is a more detailed description of the HHS Checklist:

DIGESTIVE DIFFICULTIES

1. **Belching --** This is a result of lowered digestive functions caused by the HHS.
2. **Bloating --** This feels like a spare tire under the rib cage. It occurs when food is improperly digested, and

there is a lack of hydrochloric acid which causes fullness.

3.   **Sensitivity at the waist** -- In some instances the HHS sufferer can't bear anything tight around the waist due to the sensitivity of the skin.

4.   **Intestinal gas** -- When the HHS occurs, hydrochloric acid is lowered, digestive ability is reduced, and the process of improper digestion produces putrefaction of foods in the large intestines.

5.   **Regurgitation** -- Food will stop part-way down to the stomach, sometimes with great distress, or food already ingested will come back up into the esophagus causing burning pain. This is referred to as acid reflux **or** esophageal reflux in modern medical literature.

6.   **Hiccups** -- I have never seen a case of hiccups that was not equated with the HHS. The nerve that controls the diaphragm, the phrenic nerve, starts pulsing quicker than usual and causes the diaphragm to contract sometimes violently. I have seen hiccups disappear when the stomach is gently adjusted into place.

7.   **Lack or limitation of appetite** -- Because the stomach is pushed up, this allows only a small amount of food to be received into the stomach at a time. About two hours after eating, the person will feel hungry again. Since the digestive enzymes are reduced when the HHS is present, even small amounts of food are not properly digested. See Diagram #1).

8.   **Nausea** -- As a result of altered acid levels in the stomach, because of the HHS, many sensitive individuals experience nausea with or without the presence of food in the stomach.

9.   **Vomiting** -- because of excessive acidity, due to HHS interference, the phrenic nerve produces spasms in the diaphragm accompanied by spasms produced in the stomach; the result is an expulsion of food contents from the stomach.

Diagram #1

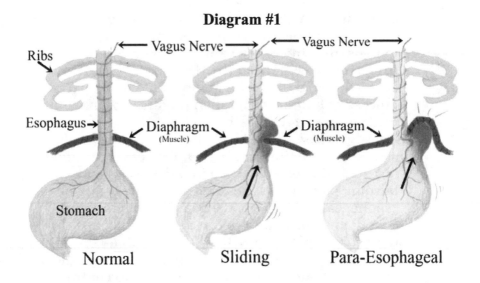

Ribs

Esophagus →

← Vagus Nerve → ← Vagus Nerve →

← Diaphragm →
(Muscle)

← Diaphragm →
(Muscle)

Stomach

Normal   Sliding   Para-Esophageal

10. **Diarrhea** -- Peristaltic action is increased as a result of the contraction in the stomach produced by the HHS. This leads to excessive and rapid evacuation of waste products.

11. **Constipation** -- Although many reasons exist for this problem, I find that when the HHS is corrected often constipation is alleviated.

12. **Colic in children** -- As with diarrhea in an adult, the condition known as "colic" is often relieved by simply correcting the HHS.

Diagram #2

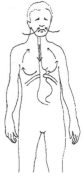

BREATHING AND CIRCULATION PROBLEMS

13. **Deep breathing curtailed** -- (See Diagram #2.) *Note that as much as two-thirds of our normal deep breathing capacity may be reduced by the HHS.*

14. **Overall fatigue and exhaustion** -- The ascended stomach (HHS) reduces the amount of breathing capacity, therefore, oxygen flow. Lack of oxygen in the tissues creates an acidic condition throughout the body which leads to enervation.

15. **Tendency to swallow air** -- This is an observed phenomenon, although not fully understood. By

swallowing air, attempt is made subconsciously to force the stomach down.

16. **Allergies** -- The HHS interferes with adrenal gland function. Proper adrenal function is necessary to prevent all types of allergic responses.

17. **Dry tickling cough** -- This is a reflex that is triggered in the throat area when the stomach is forced upward.

18. **Full feeling at base of throat** -- This is caused when the stomach crowds the esophagus.

19. **Pain or burning in upper chest** -- When these darting types of pain occur, usually after a heavy meal, at first a heart condition may be suspected. Sometimes these pains are confused with angina pectoralis. Refer to the chapter on Heart Problems.

20. **Pressure in the chest** -- The HHS presses against the lungs, reducing oxygen intake. This also can be mistaken for the beginning of angina. (See Diagram #2.)

21. **Pain in the left side of chest**-- Caused by gas being forced into chest cavity by the ascended stomach.

22. **Heartburn** -- The result of partial food reflux because of the HHS.

23. **Pressure below breastbone** -- Certain indication that the HHS is present.

24. **Lung pain** -- This symptom is rare, but it is the result of the structural interference caused by ascended stomach and reduced oxygen intake. It occurs in certain people with chest problems.

25. **Rapid heartbeat** -- Acceleration comes when the stomach crowds the heart space, pressing it against the rib cage. This usually accompanies mild anxiety.

26. **Rapid rise in blood pressure** -- Because of HHS interference, the vagus nerve is pinched at stomach level; correspondingly, the vagus branch to the heart is agitated, producing a rise in blood pressure, and, or cardiac arrhythmias.

STRUCTURAL COMPLAINTS

27. **Left shoulder pain, pain in left arm, pain in the left side of neck** -- From clinical observations, these are referral pains that disappear when the HHS is corrected.

28. **Right shoulder pain** -- Again, these are referral pains although occurring with less frequency than left

shoulder pain.

29.   **Pain between the shoulder blades** -- A dull nagging to occasionally sharp pain will occur in the center of the back between the shoulders.

30.   **Joint pain in extremities** -- If there are no structural changes indicated by X-ray, the HHS may indeed be a contributing factor and create arthritic tendencies (See chapter on Arthritis.)

31.   **Localized or overall spinal pain** -- Pain in mid-back, around and along the ribs to the back of mid-spine, in lower back, and all over spinal pain are clear evidences of HHS and are fully addressed in the chapter on Backaches.

32.   **Headaches** -- Many headaches occur because of digestive and structural disorders brought on by the HHS.

33.   **Temporo-Mandibular Joint pain (TMJ)** -- This is usually considered a dental problem. Most of the time it is, but the HHS sometimes refers pain to this area (See discussion in TMJ chapter).

34.   **Bruxism** (Grinding of the teeth in sleep) -- There is strong evidence that the HHS is involved.

STRESS

35.   **Dizziness** -- This can occur from lack of oxygen to the brain, because the stomach interferes with the lung's ability to inhale deeply.

36.   **Mental confusion** -- The HHS creates a low blood sugar situation and in certain individuals affects mental clarity.

37.   **Shakiness** -- When the HHS occurs, the blood sugar situation which results can cause shakiness.

38.   **Anxiety attacks** -- An almost prevailing symptom of the HHS. The more serious and prolonged the condition, the more likely the progression from light anxiety to a full-blown anxiety attack. The HHS is a major linking factor here.

39.   **Insomnia** -- When lying flat on back, the stomach will ascend during and sometimes before sleep, causing distress and anxiousness that can interfere with sleep.

40.   **Hyperactivity in children** -- The HHS interferes with adrenal gland function. In young children when adrenal

16

glands are over-stimulated, it can create a situation of excessive hyperactivity.

OTHER AILMENTS

41. **Craving for sugar or alcohol --** See chapters on Hypoglycemia and Alcoholism.
42. **Candida Albicans --** See chapter on Candida Albicans.
43. **Menstrual or Prostate Trouble --** See chapters on Prostate and Premenstrual Syndrome.
44. **Urinary difficulties - -** See chapter on Kidneys.
45. **Hoarseness- -** See chapter on Hoarseness.
46. **Obesity --** See chapter on Obesity.

Chapter 3

IMPORTANCE OF THE VAGUS NERVE

The vagus nerve is the basic factor involved in the distresses caused by the hiatal hernia. It extends throughout the body, is so diverse in function, and reaches so many glands and organs that it has been nicknamed "the wanderer." Envision the comprehensive effect when this nerve's function is disrupted. There is interference of the vagus if the stomach is only slightly displaced. It doesn't belong above the diaphragm, even a quarter of an inch. It is the vagus nerve that largely controls the production of hydrochloric acid, which is of paramount importance in the initial digestion of food. If this nerve is pinched by a hiatal hernia the acid is reduced, thereby causing either putrification or fermentation of foods that have been eaten, no matter how well they are combined. (See Diagram #5.)

Hydrochloric acid (HCL) is the only form of acid that is beneficial to the body. Other waste products, mostly protein in origin, that have a tendency to accumulate within the tissues of a healthy person form harmful acid by-products. These are termed "tissue acid waste" or "tissue acidity." The healthy person usually has a proper amount of HCL produced by the stomach and the vagus nerve to digest and assimilate foods; therefore, these protein acid accumulations in the tissues will not interfere with normal cellular function.

Let us look at the diagram again. Any acidity in the tissues of any gland or organ will force that organ to try to maintain its own nature, which is mostly alkaline. Acidity has a smothering, irritating effect upon the tissues if out of normal balance (20% acid and 80% alkaline). This causes one to breathe quickly in an attempt to throw off the acid imbalance created by excessive vagus nerve stimulation. From the vagus nerve level of the heart, the pulse and the blood pressure

Diagram #3

PATHWAY OF THE VAGUS NERVE

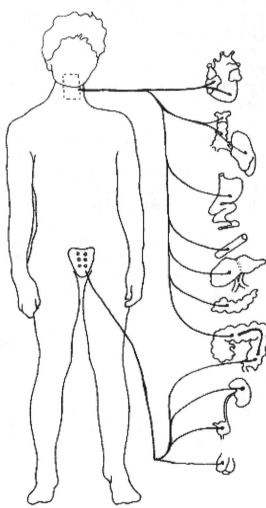

Heart

Larynx
  Bronchi & Lungs
  Esophagus

Stomach

Small Intestine

Abdominal Blood Vessels

Liver
  Gall Bladder

Pancreas

Colon
  Link Between Vagus &
  Pelvic Parasympathetic
  Rectum

Kidney

Bladder

External Genitalia

increase. The lungs are forced to breathe rapidly.

The liver and gall bladder overproduce bile and enzymes, further irritating the digestive system. The pancreas overproduces insulin, which can quickly lead to a low blood sugar episode. The small intestines can slow the production of an alkaline substance called "chyle", which leads to all becoming excessively acidic. The large intestine responds by either diarrhea or constipation. In other words, at every level a mess occurs when the vagus overproduces acidity. Multiply this condition by the number of times daily when one gets upset. Is it any wonder there are so many health problems?

The delicate stomach contracts at even the smallest negative feelings that are generated. The vagus nerve is the mainspring of our feelings. One can wind the mainspring however he wishes as long as he is aware that he is the one that's winding it. Anger, fear and jealousy lead to many biochemical changes that induce excess acidity in the body. The body expresses sickness only when it is excessively acid. The illness then expressed is the body's way of balancing this acidity.

It is vitally important to understand the ways to deal with these core level problems that cause the stomach to displace itself upwards through or against the diaphragm.

Chapter 4

ANGELA - A CASE STUDY

I am pleased to be able to offer this case study of Angela. She is a patient of mine who was willing to do whatever it takes to get the message out of just how dangerous HHS really is. She has agreed for me to use pictures and personal information about the history of her case to demonstrate how easy it is to miss this monstrous syndrome. The case as it is presented is as true to her memory as possible, and there is no exaggeration in this story. So many people are mistreated by medical and alternative practitioners when it comes to this tricky problem that I feel it is necessary to elaborate in some detail about the events. Much of this story is in her words. I have seen about fifty cases that approached this level of seriousness and thousands of others who were suffering in lesser degrees.

Angela remembers having anxiety attacks, accompanied by shortness of breath and appetite loss since she was twelve years old. Although this did not happen on a regular basis, it was mostly the result of stressful situations. Starting in college these attacks occurred more frequently, approximately once every two weeks.

When I first examined and questioned Angela, she was having a severe anxiety attack with shortness of breath from a highly stressful situation that had occurred earlier that day. She reported that over the last six months she had experienced a large number of symptoms, though she did not tell me that she had been medically diagnosed with a hiatal hernia on the first visit. She had been to eight different doctors to seek relief. Among these were two doctors of internal medicine, one pulmonary specialist (lungs), a rheumatologist, two general practitioners, and two emergency room doctors.

To show the reader the severity of what she experienced, this section is her story in her words.

"It all began in the summer of 2005. I have always been a very energetic and outgoing person, having enough energy to go from daylight until dark. During this summer I found myself feeling extremely tired and lifeless. I would have to force myself out of bed and by the end of the day; I was ready to collapse. I started noticing my anxiety and shortness of breath worsen. My lips would stay chapped and no matter the temperature, I stayed cold all the time. For no apparent reason, my hands would start to shake, my breathing would become very shallow, and a numbness which started in my stomach would make its way to my limbs.

It was at this time that I sought help from my doctor regarding these symptoms. Upon my physician's first examination, she suspected I had lupus. She explained that it would cause extreme fatigue and would affect the entire body. Although my test showed low white blood cell count, my doctor could not determine for certain that lupus was the problem. She suggested that I get more rest, start on multi-vitamins, and follow up if these symptoms did not cease. Over the next few weeks, the symptoms increased with my anxiety and tiredness worsening day by day. I developed a severe sore throat one night in late September which caused me to go to the Emergency Room. It was the ER doctor that found that I had contracted mononucleosis. I felt so relieved that these symptoms were finally named. It had been so discouraging, feeling my health decline daily, and not knowing what was wrong. I felt confident that after I got over the mono, I would begin feeling like my old self again. Unfortunately, that did not happen.

Over the next few months my existing symptoms worsened, and I began a steady decline. That winter I completely lost my appetite, losing over 30 pounds. I had no energy; my hands shook all the time, and the numbness which before had been an occasional happening stayed in my stomach all the time. My system was depleted from October to March. I battled with mono, bronchitis, pneumonia, sinusitis and intestinal problems. I was referred to several specialists, and going to the doctor became a weekly event. Although I was doing everything I could to find relief, my condition only became worse. None of these doctors could pinpoint the problem, merely treating me for viruses and bacteria and prescribing more medication. At the time of my first severe attack, I was taking a half dozen prescriptions including Levaquin, Advair Inhaler, Phenegren, Lomotil, Naproxen,

Lexapro, Adivan and Acidophilus and multi-vitamins.

The day of this attack I could feel myself getting very anxious throughout the day. My shaking became worse, and my breathing very labored. My hands felt numb and began to draw inward, with my fingers touching. My feet pulled toward each other. There was a tingling in my mouth, causing speech to be difficult. My eyes closed, and I could not force them open. I felt that I had no control over my body; yet, during this time I was still conscious and alert.

When the emergency room doctors could find nothing physically wrong; they concluded my condition was all in my head and wanted to commit me to a mental institution. It was not until several hours later that these crippling symptoms eased, and I felt that I could breathe and had control again. When I was referred to the rheumatologist, I was experiencing excruciating pain in every joint. In addition, I had extreme shortness of breath, and was in so much pain that I had tears streaming down my face. The doctor who saw me said that he also thought I had some sort of mental problem. He suggested that I seek counseling because he could see nothing wrong. I received no answers from all these doctors; yet, my health declined daily.

At this time, I was aware my mental state was in disarray. I knew I was I sick; however, after extensive testing and there were no conclusive answers, I felt depressed and that I was fighting a losing battle. Even my friends reported that I had terrible mood swings, which I had never had before.

I had two more attacks after this; the second of which came after I met Dr. Baroody. He had already found a Hiatal Hernia; however, there were so many conditions when he first started working with me that the Hernia did not seem to be the primary cause at the time. I visited him one afternoon while the attack was already in great progress. As before, my mouth was tingling and beginning to draw. My hands were completely pulled together, and I was gasping for breath. I was in terrible pain in all my joints and, once again, was to the point of tears. He suggested that he adjust my stomach first to see if the correction would eliminate any of these symptoms. Within fifteen minutes of his adjusting my stomach, **ALL MY SYMPTOMS CEASED.** I was AMAZED! Immediately, I could breathe again; the pain in my joints disappeared; the numbness left. My hands and mouth returned to normal within minutes. I felt more relief in those fifteen minutes than I had in seven months. I actually felt hungry for the first time in months. I started smiling again. All the tiredness left out of my muscles, and I was NO PAIN!"

Following is the list of symptoms Angela exhibited when she came for her first visit. You will notice that she has most of the symptoms from the Hiatal Hernia Checklist with many new ones added. When she states she was symptom-free after I pulled the stomach into place, she is referring to the multitude of immediate symptoms. In particular, I watched as her hands and feet unwound, straightened and returned to normal. The more long-term symptoms from years of HHS disruption began resolving over the next two weeks. When the stomach is in place and the vagus nerve is no longer pinched, healing accelerates for the more compromised complex biochemical pathways.

I think it is noteworthy to mention that her internal medicine doctors had found a hiatal hernia but told her the same story I have heard a thousand times: "You have a small hiatal hernia, but it could not possibly be the cause of all these symptoms. ***BESIDES, ALMOST EVERYONE HAS A HIATAL HERNIA. GO ON AND DON'T WORRY ABOUT IT."*** (emphasis mine)

- Bloating
- Sensitivity at the waist
- Intestinal gas
- Hiccup
- Lack or limitation of appetite
- Nausea
- Vomiting
- Diarrhea
- Constipation
- Deep breathing curtailed
- Overall fatigue and exhaustion
- Tendency to swallow air
- Allergies
- Dry tickling cough
- Full feeling at base of throat
- Pain or burning in upper chest
- Pressure in the chest
- Pain in the left side of chest
- Heartburn
- Pressure below breastbone
- Lung pain
- Very rapid heartbeat
- Rise in blood pressure, but still low
- Left shoulder pain, pain in left arm, pain in left side of neck
- Right shoulder pain
- Pain between the shoulder blades
- Joint pain in extremities
- Localized or overall spinal pain

- Headaches
- TMJ -Temporo-Mandibular Joint pain
- Pain behind and in both ears
- Dizziness
- Shakiness
- Mental confusion
- Anxiety attacks
- Insomnia
- Craving for salt and vinegar
- Menstrual problems
- Urinary difficulties
- Hoarseness
- Stayed cold all the time, no matter what the temperature
- Severe mood swings from manic to depressive to obsessive
- Discolored bowel movements (one day black, one day green.)
- Hair loss (It fell out by the handfuls)
- Diagnosed hypoglycemia
- Heaviness at the stomach level (at the xiphoid process)
- Numbness in mouth and extremities
- Inability to open the eyes while still conscious and able to talk
- Severely chapped lips
- Inward contractions of hands
- Inward contractions of feet
- Downward contraction of the head toward the chest
- Overall contracted fetal position
- Pursing of the lips
- Inability to sit or stand, even for a short period
- Severe coccyx pain
- Extreme sensitivity to any touch, no matter how light (such as a hand or bed sheet caused pain and crying)
- Cry very easily
- Grayish skin color
- Occasional lifeless looking stare

25

Angela #1
(During Full HHS Attack)

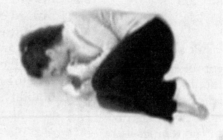

Angela #2
(Hand Position During Attack)

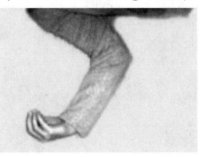

Angela #3
(Feet Position During Attack)

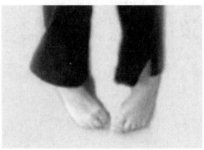

THE RESULTS OF
HIATAL HERNIA
SYNDROME
IMBALANCES

Chapter 5

OVERALL DIGESTION IMBALANCES

The first part of Chapter 4 summarizes how the basic digestive processes are disrupted by the HHS.

The second part consists of the technical facts and is optional if your focus is mainly on the conditions the HHS. I have offered my opinion in certain areas. My conclusions stem from a great deal of research and observation over a twenty-year period. It details some of the more important physiological workings of the digestive system as they relate to the vagus nerve and the HHS. Read Part II at your discretion. Hopefully, it will offer some additional ideas about the complexity of this syndrome and why it is so difficult to diagnose and rebalance.

PART I

The HHS so strongly affects the various stages of digestion that its presence leads to many major illnesses. Once digestion is affected, food is either improperly assimilated or not at all. This causes the body to look for food within itself and starts the processes of bone demineralization (osteoarthritis), because the body needs calcium which it is not absorbing.

This is just the beginning of what can happen. Next, the endocrine glands become sluggish. The most important of these are the adrenal and thyroid glands. The adrenal glands provide us with our energy and help to regulate blood sugar levels. The thyroid keeps the body at the right rate of balance, neither too fat nor sluggish nor too thin and overly excitable. When the food they need is not properly digested these glands under-function from lack of nutritional support. Then the body develops low blood sugar syndromes, premenstrual syndromes, and bowel problems. This cycle can continue for years, depending on one's personal body chemistry. This creates degeneration by increasingly devastating degrees, which finally takes the form of severe allergies, a constant flu because of lowered immune function, diabetes, or even death-producing problems.

We are looking for the beginning point. My own research leads me to the stomach and digestive disruption. This would point us to the Hiatal Hernia Syndrome as a possible culprit.

Perhaps the HHS started as a purely emotionally stressful situation, or it may have been induced by a mechanical injury. Regardless, it seems that we find ourselves at the same crossroads: the HHS stays up and the vicious cycle of improper assimilation predisposes the various problems discussed in the later chapters.

PART II

These are the technical facts: Digestion begins as salivary amylase mixes with food. A bolus, which is a combination of the chewed food and salivary enzymes, is formed. This bolus of food is swallowed to the Lower

Diagram #4

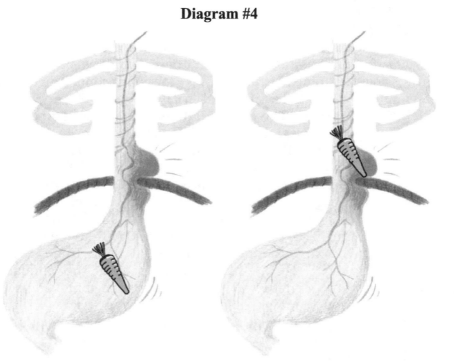

Undigested food due to HHS   **Food blocked due to HHS**

Esophageal Sphincter (LES). Should even the smallest amount of stomach ascension occur here, the LES may malfunction.

This in itself would stop the bolus from entry into the fundus of the stomach. (See Diagram #4) The commonly reported symptom of pain and tightness to the side, (sometimes exactly inferior to the xyphoid process) is one of the first signs of stomach ascension and LES involvement. We are faced here with several problems occurring simultaneously. Not only are the lungs compromised which makes breathing more shallow, but the heart is also affected. This often leads to anxiety symptoms because the heart starts into tachycardia, and breathing becomes even more shallow and rapid. This can perpetuate an increase in pulse rate and blood pressure. To further complicate the problem, the adrenal products epinephrine -- norepinephrine, enter the bloodstream in quantities as high as 1 part per million. This is the body's attempt to deal with the stresses of the HHS. Unless the stomach returns to its normal position, there could be a possibility of a true anxiety attack.

In some cases, a damaging cardiac episode could occur. Assuming the person has no cardiac history, the heart is in no immediate danger from HHS interference. If the HHS has been ongoing for many years, however, there could be progressive cardiovascular disease occurring from improper digestion causing elevated cholesterol and triglyceride levels and poor calcium absorption. The accumulation of these substances in the arteries could precipitate a cardiac episode.

One of several things could happen to cause stomach ascension. The person may become over-stressed from work, family, emotions, recreation or an accident. Any of these can be enough to trigger the parasympathetic portion of the vagus nerve extending into the stomach. This stimulation causes gastric secretion at an undesirable time and initiates a spastic reaction in the smooth muscles of the stomach from excess hydrochloric acid (HCL). The result is that the stomach pushes upward. There will be either a very minor muscle involvement or a major insult (tear) to the tissue of the diaphragmatic esophageal hiatus. Consequently, a larger portion of the stomach could ascend through the diaphragm and be closer to the heart.

The function of the vagus nerve changes, after the stomach has ascended, by either a stressful episode or a mechanical trauma. One would think this could produce an oversecretion of hydrochloric acid (HCL); however, the opposite occurs.

If there is an HHS involvement and our chewed food enters the stomach, it creates definite reduction in the breakdown of the food bolus in the initial digestive phase. Two of the three phases of gastric secretions are under vagal control. These are the cephalic (first phase), gastric (second phase). I suspect the intestinal or third phase, though not usually described as having vagal involvement, has an indirect effect through the enterogastric reflex. Vagal control continues as the food enters the small intestine. In fact, the vagus itself has a branch all the way into the midway of the colon!

In the gastric phase, antral distension causes both secretion of pepsinogen and hydrochloric acid. If the vagus is impinged, the stimulation caused by distension to the receptors in the gastric mucosa that normally initiate reflexes of afferent and efferent vagal fiber will also begin under-functioning. To what degree can antral distension occur if the stomach is ascended? If the vagus is impinged, the production of acetylcholine (the most potent stimulus for pepsinogen production) is thereby reduced. This means a reduction in gastrin, which means a further reduction in hydrochloric acid production.

Thus, the action of hydrochloric acid (HCL) is paramount. It can denature proteins, break chemical bonds, help activate pepsinogen, inactivate salivary amylase, and even act as an effective disinfectant.

What happens as a result of improper breakdown of chyme by under-secretion of hydrochloric acid? This requires consideration of pancreatic secretion and its delivery of digestive enzymes. Pancreatic secretion increases in response to vagal stimulation. Even the stimuli that cause pancreatic secretion by the presence of food in the mouth are subject to the reflex pathways in the vagus nerve. Again, if the vagus nerve energies are reduced, production of pancreatic juices is also diminished. The major factors in the control of pancreatic secretion are hormonal and involve secretin and cholecystokinin (CCK). The argument here is that if hydrochloric acid production is lessened, then not as much secretin will be produced since the presence of hydrochloric acid in the duodenum or small intestine causes the production of secretin.

Let us go back a step and look at what occurs when too

31

much acid is produced via vagal stimulation by emotional stress. When the HHS is present and food is eaten, the bolus passes the pyloric sphincter with a backwash of excess hydrochloric acid. In some patients an X-ray of the pyloric area may appear calcified, since so much excess acid has passed this area. Upon closer examination, it may be found that this is an acidification instead. The improperly broken down bolus enters as chyme into the duodenum. The bile that would normally emulsify the broken down chyme is not able to do so properly because of the larger particles. This causes a backwash of bile into the pylorus and into the fundus of the stomach, irritating the mucosal stomach lining and causing the parietal cells to produce more hydrochloric acid in an attempt to bring homeostasis (body balance). This excess acid is secreted where no food bolus exists for it to act upon and where the mucosal lining is already in a weakened and irritated state. The HCL then creates a burning lesion of ulceration. Because smooth muscle contracts when too much hydrochloric acid is produced on an empty stomach, there is acid reflux which easily bypasses the already affected lower esophageal sphincter. The person is then diagnosed as having reflux esophagitis.

Since the pancreas and liver both are partially under vagal control and the vagus is impinged, there is a definite reduction and delivery of proper enzyme control. Digestion is further affected and the person may exhibit a subclinical-level of malnourishment.

It is not my intent here to discuss spinal involvement in detail; however, it is important to note that nerves coming from the spine affect the body in direct relationship to individual ability to function at optimum level.

Recent research on the impingement of the sciatic nerve in rats has indicated a 60% reduction in nerve impulse along the nerve axis in three minutes. If this is true, the theory of nerve impingement's having a significant effect on its targeted organ function must be re-evaluated. Then, let us look at nerve impingement at the spinal level as a probability.

The liver produces bile. When there are errant signals to the liver through the pinching of the 9th thoracic nerve root, we find an overproduction of bile. The mechanism that controls bile formation is affected. With too much bile production we see a loop of problems occurring between the small intestine and the liver via the enterohepatic circulation. As more bile pours into the small intestines, it is reabsorbed via the portal vein back into the liver signaling that more bile production is unnecessary. Further, as too much bile enters the small intestine the available fats are not given a chance to be coated and form chylomicrons.

Triglyceride formations become too heavy; they backup into the liver via the portal vein, cause fat accumulation which congests the liver even further, and cause more triglycerides to enter the system. Looking at the vagus nerve again, we find that disturbance with this nerve causes an underproduction of chyle in the small intestine, which would further add to improper chylomicron production. Assuming the vagus is functioning properly, the smooth muscle in the wall of the gall bladder will contract upon vagal stimulation. We have an excess amount of bile being formed in the liver and released into the small intestine, then looped back for more production via the enterohepatic circulation. What is happening to the gall bladder? It fills too fast; then gallstones and gravel result.

Problems with excessive bile and poorly digested food, complicated by vagal interference all the way down the tract, finally end in the large intestine. Constipation or diarrhea usually occurs in these cases.

Constipation is seen for two reasons. One is that food not properly digested in the small intestine moves slowly through the colon. Second, the vagus nerve branch to the large intestine could be under-functioning as a result of its initial pinching in the upper stomach. Then, a more serious problem occurs here. As the fecal matter resides in the intestinal wall, water is reabsorbed back into the body, and the rich blood vessels near this absorbing organ are filled with toxic distillates from the large intestine. This overloads the liver, as the liver tries to purify the blood. This causes another hindrance to digestive enzyme activity. Since liver function is further interrupted, the production of lymph is reduced and the overall waste disposal system is slowed down at the cellular tissue level. This plays hand in hand with yet more constipation, the possibility of diverticulosis and other bowel-related problems.

What about vagotomy -- the cutting of the vagus nerve branch into the stomach? The vagus is quite extensive and so little is known about its parasympathetic system function at this point that I doubt whether vagotomy is as effective as it appears. True, it reduces problems of high acidity, but is it necessary? If a vagotomy is performed on the upper branch of that nerve, what about the vagus connections in the duodenum? It is my contention that the vagus is being stimulated in the duodenum by the peristaltic motility of the intrinsic plexus. This loops back into the gastric phase of the fundus, whether or not the vagus is severed at the upper stomach level. It is highly conceivable that although not as much vagal stimulation is occurring at the onset of digestion, we still have the same problem - the HHS. The other symptoms still exist; the vagotomy is doing little more than dealing with excessive hydrochloric acid production. This makes matters worse, for regardless of whether or not an ulcer exists, the fact remains that hydrochloric acid is still needed to break down food and assure proper nutrition to the cells. The obvious answer is to deal with the ulcer in a different way until it is healed. If stomach ascension is corrected, it is possible that much ulceration can be avoided and rebalanced.

Another aspect of my thesis to be considered is that nerve energies are blocked and shunted by intestinal adhesions and lesions in the lacteal ducts. Again, one of the primary nerves involved here is the vagus, which is pinched at the HHS level of the upper stomach. What happens is highly significant; the seriousness of this problem is widespread.

Adhesions can be formed in the small intestine for several reasons. First, there could be an injury to the abdominal area. Such trauma significantly reduces blood flow, causing an adhesion. Secondly, the lacteal ducts will lesion, causing a smaller amount of available digestive area. The production of chyle is significantly reduced through these lesions, leaving the body with an unavailable amount of chyle to coat the triglycerides in the small intestine. Since the small intestine is also innervated by the sympathetic nervous system (splanchnic nerves), as well as the parasympathetic nervous system (vagus nerve), we see another manifestation of abnormal physiological behavior in which the smooth muscle of the jejunum and ileum can spasm. This generally unexplored manifestation is nevertheless a functional reality.

To a greater or lesser extent, I find these adhesion problems in an astounding number of patients. Who knows all the problems which these lesions in the lacteal ducts are really causing? For our purposes here we look only at adhesions and the spasms they produce in relation to the vagus, stomach (HHS), and assimilation problems. If left untreated, these spasms cause a reflex action through sympathetic innervation (splanchnic nerves) up into the rest of the body. Depending upon the extent of the lesions and the particular biochemical sensitivities of the individual afflicted, there are several possibilities. One of these is epilepsy. (See chapter on Epilepsy Imbalances.)

There are, however, less obvious possibilities. If there are adhesions in the small intestines, then there will be less surface area for digestion. This has a direct effect on chyme and the Peyer's Patches. The lacteal ducts are also affected by improper vagal stimulation. Definite disturbances in the digestion and the distribution of nutrition to the rest of the body follow.

Manifestations of this phenomenon could lead to hypoglycemia, premenstrual syndrome, and other assorted nutritional difficulties. Further, the lacteal duct lesions and adhesions may present another heretofore unsuspected danger. The reason for this is the interesting way that the small intestine aids the body in maintaining a proper acid-base relationship. I find it most surprising that acid-alkaline biochemistry is not studied in more detail as it applies to the human system. Volumes upon volumes are written dealing with the effects of proper and improper usage of acid and alkaline reactions in the soil in the whole field of agriculture; yet, little is known about these reactions within the body.

Every book you care to study on human physiology will go into the study of chylomicrons, but little is known about the effect of chyle within the human system. **Chyle is an alkalizing force within the body**. The importance of this is that the body works more efficiently when there is proper acid - alkaline balance.

When too much acidity is displayed in the body, it presents a clinical problem. Excessive tissue acidity causes glands and organs alike to under-function. This is particularly seen in diabetes.

The content of most foods in America are acid-forming after entering the system. Thus, it is easy to see how the alkalizing influence of chyle, should it be disturbed, causes a body system to move into excessive acidity. When the lacteal ducts are lesioned or adhesions exist, we observe a definite decrease of chyle production from the lacteal ducts and the Peyer's Patches.

Lesions and adhesions in the jejunum and ileum occur for one or more of these reasons:

1. The HHS causing a disturbance in vagal function, hydrochloric acid production and/or excessive bile formation.
2. A trauma to the abdominal area causing the lesion.
3. Spinal misalignment causing nerve pressures reflexing into the jejunum and ileum to cause poor circulation which leads to under-function and adhesions being formed.
4. All or any of these causes.

We still see the lack of small intestine function and underproduction of chyle which helps balance body needs.

Couple the above with a diet of poor, acid-forming, refined foods and we have a body that might express disease in any number of ways, depending upon its particular biochemical predisposition.

There is another area that warrants investigation. How does a normally functioning small intestine produce enough chyle, enter it into the system, and have such a powerful and important alkalizing effect? Current research has shown that chyle coats the triglyceride molecule and becomes a chylomicron. It is dumped into the subclavian area via the lymphatic ducts for use in circulation or storage until a time the body needs the triglyceride and releases it by the action of the adrenal hormones. A possible pathway is that chylomicrons could enter general circulation via the portal vein.

I propose a third way. Chyle enters the lymphatics by permeating the walls of the jejunum and ileum and then entering general circulation.

Who knows all the implications at this time? It is still an open field of research that may change the subsequent focus of health care, but unless research alters it, I stand by these views.

Chapter 6

INTESTINAL TRACT IMBALANCES

The incredible significance of the well-being of the large intestine or colon is that it marks the difference between a high quality life and an unhealthy one. The hiatal hernia can be greatly aggravated by a constipated or spastic colon. Intestinal gas pushes up from the inside and displaces the stomach. The slightest bit of upward protrusion of the stomach causes suffering. Equally important is the interference with the vagus nerve at this level of the stomach. (See Diagram #5)

Diagram #5

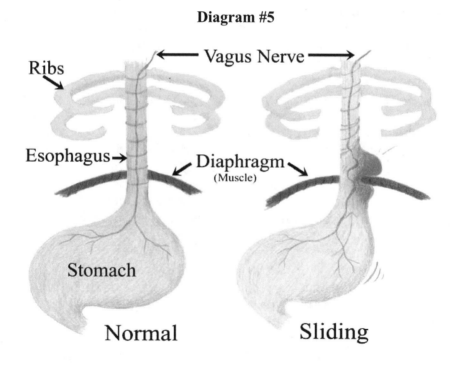

The vagus has branches directly into the colon. (See Diagram #3.) Thus, according to a person's particular biochemistry, either constipation or diarrhea results. If the vagus nerve no longer produces hydrochloric acid because it is pinched, then improperly digested food has ample time and opportunity to ferment, putrefy, and stop up the colon.

Colon cancer is our nation's # 1 cancer killer today. If 85% of the population has the Hiatal Hernia Syndrome (HHS) is there a connection? If there is even the slightest bit of constipation or diarrhea, check for its presence. Why not treat the stomach first?

In many patients, when the stomach is dropped into place, I have watched an immediate reversal of intestinal problems. With the further addition of hydrochloric acid and food enzymes to their diet, those heavy, bloated feelings also disappeared.

Consider the case of Mrs. N. who had diarrhea after every meal for many years. She had lost her appetite. A medical diagnosis of hiatal hernia was given. In surgery her gall bladder was removed and her diaphragm was repaired, which is the medical procedure for correcting the hiatal hernia. Afterwards, she had more intense pain in the stomach area and dropped from 120 pounds to 80 pounds. When she came to me, I corrected the syndrome and from that day she regained her appetite, recovered the lost weight, and started having regular bowel movements.

Irritable Bowel Syndrome (IBS) is an affliction that affects 22 million people. I have never seen its presence without finding the HHS also.

Celiac disease is a digestive disease that damages the small intestine and interferes with absorption of nutrients from food. Gluten found in wheat, oats, rye, barley, spelt, kamet and teff are to be avoided. I can see where a possible link here could come from the vagus nerve being disrupted by the HHS at the stomach level. Remember, the vagus does go into the small intestines.

Although 1 in 4,700 Americans have been diagnosed with celiac disease, a recent study suggests that the real number is closer to 1 in 250. My findings are even worse. Although my tests are kinesiological, I find about 1 in 5 with some mild to moderate disturbance that is pointing in this direction. I am not stating that this number actually has celiac disease, just a proclivity in that direction.

The human body is host to billions of microorganisms. Some of these are good guys and some are bad guys. There are more than 400 different species of bacteria in the gut alone, and who knows what number of parasites and viruses.

Leaky Gut Syndrome is a very serious issue. When the large intestines (also called the colon) leaks through the walls, many negative conditions arise. Among these are chronic food and environmental allergies, psoriasis, lowered immune function, blood sugar disorders, a build up of cancer cell toxins, chemical sensitivities, irritable bowel syndrome, chronic arthritis, Crohn's disease, hepatitis, pancreatitis and chronic fatigue.

I cannot say that Leaky Gut Syndrome is a direct result of HHS interference, but there is no doubt in my mind that it could be an indirect result. Lack of proper digestion slowly weakens the protein in all the body's viscera and this could lead to a softening of the small and/or large intestinal walls over a period of time. Even Edgar Cayce, considered the father of modern holistic medicine, spoke about the small intestines leaking poisons back into the general circulation of the body in the 1930's.

It is highly probable that prolific use of irritating laxatives would not be necessary if the HHS were corrected. I do not state that HHS actually causes constipation or any of its interrelated problems; however, I see the "insidious link," the Hiatal Hernia Syndrome, as a real possibility for these conditions. From a purely clinical standpoint, I have often found these imbalances related to HHS disruption. This, however, is only clinical observation, not true research. I do find it hard to believe they are not related if I discover them to be so, because when I rebalance the HHS and add the proper food supplements, the symptoms of these debilitating states of imbalance start to improve. After 25 years in the trenches with clients suffering from everything imaginable, I trust my findings and overwhelmingly successful results and can make these assertions with confidence despite fierce opposition.

NUTRITIONAL SUGGESTIONS FOR INTESTINAL TRACT IMBALANCES

The greater the body's electrical potential, the better one's state of health. The substances I recommend to be used consistently are chelates, aspartates, orotates and/or colloidal minerals, either powdered or liquid, a good multi-vitamin, H.H.S. formula or a betaine hydrochloride formula with digestive food enzymes. They improve the body's electrical potential in each condition. The following three recommendations should be done in every case:

1. Always make sure, as well as you know how, that the stomach is down! (Refer to the chapter: "What Can Be Done?")
2. Use natural digestive aids, such as H.H.S. Formula, Pan-Gest or some type of betaine hydrochloride formula. There are many good companies which produce quality digestives.
3. Use the diet outlined in Chapter 34.

Choose one or more of the following options for cleaning the intestines and regulating bowel movements. A higher fiber diet must be utilized, along with the elimination of all refined, processed foods, especially white flour and white sugar. Drink sufficient amounts of water daily. To calculate this, drink 1 ounce of water for every 2 pounds of body weight, e.g. a 160 lb. man should drink 80 ounces of water which equals 2 ½ quarts of water per day.

OPTIONS

1. Add a natural herbal laxative such as Can-Clear or a liquid herbal tonic.
2. Use psyllium husks. 1 tablespoon -- 2x a day in 10 oz of water. In some cases, psyllium actually constipates people. If you are one of these people, discontinue usage.
3. If you take psyllium, do not also take an herbal cleaner such as Can-Clear at the same time on a consistent basis.
4. Take some type of acidophilus product such as Colonize, 1 capsule -- 3x a day.
5. Drink a cup of Senna leaf tea before bed.
6. Take some type of aloe vera tablets or use Can-Clear - 2 before bed.
7. Fast for one day a week -- eat no food; just drink juice or water.
8. Take one tablespoon of cold-pressed castor oil for one night. After that take Can-Clear or Aloe Vera tablets each night for one week. Repeat this once a month until

regulated.

9. During the day drink two glasses of water with 1 tablespoon of Swedish Bitters.

10. Colonics are highly recommended. (Consult your holistic physician.)[1]

---

[1] These products are obtainable by the general public. The named products can be found in the mini-catalog in the back of this book. There are many companies which produce fine digestive products. Your nutritionally-minded practitioner can help you with your choice and dosages. Since these recommendations cannot be given in detail but only as guidelines, no responsibility can be taken by the author if they are abused. For further understanding and comments, refer to the many informative books available on the subject of nutrition and diet.

Chapter 7

ULCER IMBALANCES

The traditional way of thinking about ulceration does not consider the physiological mechanics from the standpoint of Hiatal Hernia Syndrome (HHS) disruption. In light of information previously given, consider some facts about what the stomach does to hydrochloric acid (HCL) and digestive enzyme function.

When food enters the upper part of the stomach, hydrochloric acid (HCL) is supposed to be stimulated and awaiting its duty of breaking down the food. The vagus nerve signals the release of most of the HCL available in the stomach. (See Diagram #6, How to Get an Ulcer) Next, the digested food goes into the duodenum. There, secreted by the gall bladder, bile is released. Bile simply makes more space between food particles for their digestion. This is an emulsifying action.

Bile is an alkaline substance. The power of an alkaline substance is often understated. For instance, Drano®, a well known commercial drain cleanser, is alkaline. If this alkaline solution is put on your finger, you can watch an interesting phenomenon. Although you will feel no pain, you will be able to slough off the top layer of skin quite easily. This is because highly alkaline substances work quickly on unprotected living tissue. Fortunately, we have a mucous lining in the stomach that somewhat protects our gut from most of the effects of excess alkalinity (bile) and acidity (HCL). (See Diagram #6)

If the stomach is up (HHS), the vagus nerve function is altered which reduces the HCL required to digest whatever food does manage to get past the esophageal sphincter. When food is not broken down by hydrochloric acid, by the time it reaches this lower part of the stomach, the amount of bile excreted by the gall bladder forms an excess. This excess bile (alkaline) substance then washes back into the top part of the stomach and sloughs off some of the valuable protective mucous lining.

Diagram #6

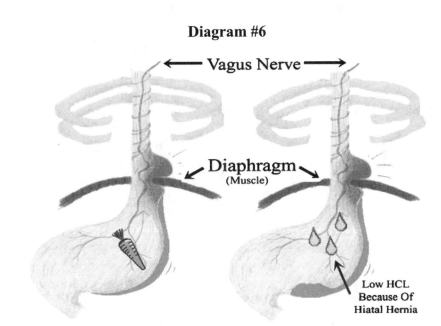

HHS causes bile to back up into stomach resulting in undigested food. Excess bile sloughs off the stomach lining. HCL increases.

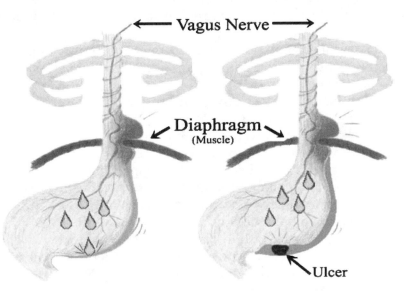

HCL burns through the weakened stomach lining. This causes an ulcer.

Remember, our bodies have a prime directive; **survival at all costs.** Part of this survival mechanism is called <u>homeostasis</u>, or the balancing of the entire system to make it work.

The stomach finds itself in a most peculiar predicament. It discovers that suddenly it has a large amount of an alkaline substance, where it is usually only accustomed to the production of acid. Again, the stomach must maintain balance, so it over-produces HCL from the parietal cells within the stomach walls to neutralize the situation. We have the already weakened or sloughed off mucous lining of the stomach by excess bile. Then hydrochloric acid pours into an unprotected empty gut. HCL is purported to have a pH of 1 or 2. This could burn a hole in the rug. That is just what it does to the poor stomach lining. It actually burns it -- in some cases all the way through -- because there is no longer any mucous lining for protection. This is called an ulceration, or just plain ulcer.

To summarize how an ulcer occurs:
1. The stomach goes up -- HHS.
2. This interferes with hydrochloric acid (HCL) production by way of the vagus nerve.
3. Some food may be blocked from entry into the stomach creating discomfort and pain just above the stomach. (See Diagram #4).
4. The food that does enter the stomach is not properly broken down by HCL.
5. The food goes into the lower stomach where alkaline bile is produced.
6. This bile washes back into the upper stomach and sloughs off some of the mucous (protective layer there.)
7. The parietal cells produce an excess of HCL in an attempt to balance out the excess alkalinity (bile.)
8. This excess HCL then causes an irritated lesion in the area where the mucous is no longer there to protect it and no food is present to slow it down. **RESULT: ULCER.**

HELICOBACTER PYLORI

Helicobacter pylori is a spiral-shaped bacterium that lives in the stomach and has a special way of adapting to the highly acidic environment. It was initially discovered in the 1892 and has had a long history of rediscoveries. The most recent was in 1983 in Perth, Australia, where its role in stomach problems was made clearly evident. It has been studied extensively and believed by the medical community to play an important role in the development of gastritis and peptic ulcers.

There has been a shift in mainstream ulcer care from the widespread use of antacids, which temporarily alleviated some symptoms but did nothing to address the root cause of the problem. Potent antibiotics are used to kill H. pylori. The results of this approach, however, have been mixed.

The inside of the stomach is bathed in about half a gallon of gastric juice every day. Gastric juice is composed of digestive enzymes and concentrated hydrochloric acid, which tear apart the toughest food or microorganism. Bacteria, viruses, and eaten foods are all consumed in this low pH environment. It was previously thought that the stomach contained no bacteria and was sterile, but Helicobacter pylori proved that wrong.

The stomach is protected from its own gastric juice by a thick layer of mucus that covers the stomach lining. Helicobacter pylori can survive and thrive by living in this mucus lining. It is able to combat the stomach acid that does reach it with an enzyme called <u>urease</u>. Urease converts urea into bicarbonate and ammonia, which are strong bases. This makes a group of acid-neutralizing chemicals around the H. pylori, protecting it from the acid in the stomach. The body's natural defenses cannot reach the bacterium in the mucus lining of the stomach. The immune system responds by sending white cells, killer T cells, and other infection fighting agents. These potential H. pylori destroyers cannot reach the infection, because they are not able to easily get through stomach lining. What is worse is that they do not go away either. The immune response grows and grows. Polymorphs die and dump their destructive compounds, called <u>superoxide radicals,</u> on stomach lining cells. Extra nutrients are then sent to reinforce the white cells. The present H. pylori feed on these. Within a short period, gastritis can result and perhaps eventually a peptic ulcer. According to one source, it may not be H. pylori itself which causes peptic ulcer, but the inflammation of the stomach lining in response to H. pylori.

H. pylori and its effects on the human body are still not well understood. While promoting the use of a combination of two or more strong antibiotics to get rid of H. pylori, doctors still cannot explain why only a small portion of those "infected" with these bacteria ever develop even a single peptic ulcer, while the vast majority of these "infected" individuals fail to develop any symptoms whatsoever. In some countries, as much as 90 percent of the population is "infected" with H. pylori, yet the frequency of gastritis and peptic ulcer disease in these countries is rather limited. The mechanisms of H. pylori transmission and spreading have not been ascertained, either. Nobody seems to know for sure how these bacteria spread from one person to the next. It appears they transmit orally by waste food and water contaminants.

As far as natural treatment goes, research shows that lactobacillus and colostrum products can have a minor effect on H. pylori. They do not eradicate it, however. Certainly, it is possible to control the symptoms caused by H. pylori with several effective natural agents. Since most of the world has this bacterial strain, and it is increasing exponentially, one has to wonder why such a large majority of those affected show no symptoms. In my own clinical experience, I have found the HHS present every time I worked on anyone who had a medically diagnosed case of H. pylori.

The HHS may be one of the initial factors which weakens the stomach and immune defenses over a period of time and allows a person who becomes exposed to H. pylori to fall victim to its ability to ensconce itself in the stomach lining.

Does the HHS cause this whole process? Yes and no. It is clearly a causative factor and it may create the path for all the other related physiological processes to go awry. I am stating that it could be the "mother of the problem" that sets up a potential ulceration, with or without the presence of H. pylori.

NUTRITIONAL SUGGESTIONS FOR ULCER IMBALANCE

1. Always make sure, as well as you know how, that the stomach is down! (Refer to chapter 34: "What Can Be Done?")
2. Use the diet outlined in Chapter 34.
3. Until all burning stops either before, during or after meals, use H.H.S. formula or a similar formula from a

46

company of your choice. Feel free to take H.H.S. Formula anytime in-between meals, particularly if there is burning. This formula will increase digestion and support the healing of ulceration. No statements about the effectiveness of this food substance on H. pylori are being made. Take at least 2 to 3 HHS Formula per meal and anytime in-between.

4. Dr. Robert Down's Original Formula: 1 part aloe vera juice and 1 part papaya juice mixed 50/50 with sugar-free ginger ale or club soda. Sip all through the day. Do not gulp!

5. Cayenne pepper capsules (old formula for ulcerations).

6. Aloe Vera juice - anytime burning starts.

For possible H. pylori infections, add the following:

1. Infect-Away -- 2 caps. 3 times a day.

2. Colonize -- 3 caps. 3 times a day.

3. Bee Powerful -- 3 caps. 2 times a day.

4. Siberian pine nut oil -- 2 to 3 teaspoons a day.

Note: *After trying natural alternatives with no results, I highly suggest you consult your doctor and start on the prescribed treatment regimen for H. pylori. This infection can be very stubborn and may only respond to medical intervention.*

Chapter 8

GALL BLADDER IMBALANCES

We are often confronted with problems related to the gall bladder. One of the most common operations done today is removal of this organ. Sometimes there is definite justification for this surgery, and in these cases it should be done. You can live without a gall bladder and if it is too diseased, I have never seen anything help much. The pain of a badly imbalanced gall bladder can be unbearable. Many times, however, I find that patients complain of exactly the same symptoms *after* the gall bladder is removed. My findings are that the HHS (the mother problem) was never addressed beforehand, and now the symptoms return with a vengeance.

Let's go back a moment to look at what happens in the upper part of the stomach. The stomach moves out of place (up), and the function of the vagus nerve is compromised. The vagus nerve also branches into the liver; simultaneously that organ starts malfunctioning. There is further involvement in the spinal area around what is called the 9th thoracic vertebrae. The nerve coming from this area of the back goes to the liver. We now have two nerves that are "pinched" and under-functioning - the vagus and the nerve from the mid-lower back area.

Bile is a substance that is made in the liver. All the gall bladder does is store the bile and release it at the right times for fat digestion. Bile is like detergent; it breaks up fat molecules into smaller pieces for better digestion by the small intestine. The small intestine absorbs and digests food, then sends nutrients back to the liver by way of the portal vein and the liver distributes these digested nutrients into the bloodstream.

What happens when something interferes with the production of bile? What if the fat you eat, which the bile is supposed to break into smaller pieces, has not first been broken down in the stomach? (See Diagram #7) This is where the HHS comes into action. Because the vagus nerve is pinched and is not supplying the right amount of hydrochloric acid for the system, the food eaten is not being digested and broken down properly. When it is the bile's turn to flow, the system is still too blocked with poorly digested food to signal the gall bladder for more bile.

You can imagine what happens next. The bile backs up

Diagram #7

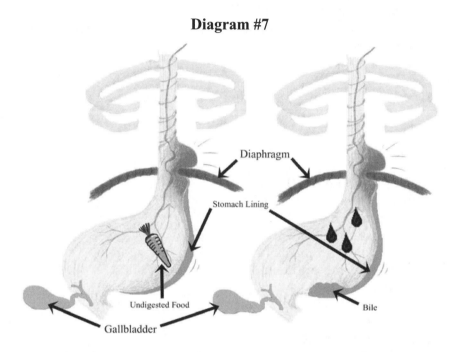

in the gall bladder and eventually starts to inflame it and to form two different kinds of gallstones. The first type is a soft green sludge that can form into hundreds of balls ranging in size from a sesame seed to a golf ball. The next type is the hard, round, whitish calcium type. These are the ones seen on an ultrasound.

It is important to understand that I am not stating that the HHS is responsible for all gall bladder problems; however it could be the link. Further, it is my opinion that if the HHS is present and goes uncorrected, the gall bladder problem will remain or recur.

Nutritional Suggestions For Gall Bladder Imbalances

1) Always make sure, as well as you know how, that the stomach is down! (Refer to the chapter: "What Can Be Done?")
2) Use natural digestive aids, particularly H.H.S. Formula, Pan-Gest or betaine hydrochloride. Use the diet outline in Chapter 34.
3) Use hot castor oil packs on the gall bladder area for 30 minutes each day.

Daily

1) Lecithin -- two tablespoons with meals.
2) Choline and Inositol--500 mg. each.
3) Biotin -- 25 mg.
4) Vitamin A -- 25,000 IU (beta carotene.)
5) Vitamin C -- 1000 mg.
6) Linseed oil -- 1000 mg.
7) Vitamin D -- 1000 IU.
8) Vitamin K-- 100 mg.
9) Vitamin E-- 600 IU.
10) Avoid all animal fat, fried foods, spicy foods, margarine, and commercial cooking oils.
11) Eat no fats!
12) Fifty percent of your diet should be juiced or raw foods.
13) Do not overeat.
14) Eat cottage cheese and/or yogurt daily.
15) Eat beets (raw or cooked).
16) Eat asparagus (cooked only), or use Aspara-Can (9 a day)
17) Fennel Seed Caps -- 1 cap. - 3x a day.
18) Cholacol 2 (from Standard Process)
19) A.F. Betafood (Standard Process).

Long Term

Gall Bladder Flush

Either:

1) Day One -- Drink one-half to one gallon of apple juice or cider, fresh or unpasteurized, if possible.
2) Day Two -- Repeat. (On both days eat nothing.)

3) Day Three -- Upon arising drink 3 ounces of apple juice. One hour later drink 4 ounces of olive oil and 4 ounces of lemon juice.

OR

1) Drink one gallon of apple juice during the course of one full day.
2) That night at 7:00 PM, take an herbal laxative.
3) At 8:00 PM, drink 4 ounces of olive oil followed by 4 ounces of lemon juice.
4) Go to bed and lie on your right side.
5) Usually, in the early morning you will have a bowel movement, and these soft green stones will be easily visible. On rare occasions, some of the hard, whitish calcium stones will come out.
6) A colonic is recommended the next day to clean out the remaining debris.

The apple juice softens the gall bladder sludge, and the olive oil and lemon juice allows almost all of the soft and sometimes even the hard stones to release into the colon. The hard stones are definitely more difficult to remove in this manner, but it is possible. There is usually a large number of green soft stone sludge that is expelled. You may see them at your next bowel movement.

Chapter 9

KIDNEY IMBALANCES

The kidneys are vital. The Chinese consider them as the seat of our life energies. When these wonderful organs malfunction even slightly, many problems occur. I find water retention in the hands and feet, pain in the mid-lower and lower back, pain from kidney stones (mostly acute) and general infection in many patients who display kidney imbalances.

The Hiatal Hernia Syndrome (HHS) is related to kidney problems in two ways. First, when the HHS is occurring, the stress control system, the adrenal glands, are affected. (See Chapter: Adrenal Gland Imbalances) The kidneys are influenced by the adrenals. Thus, if those glands are under-producing, the kidneys are lowered in function.

Second, the pelvic nerve is directly affected by the vagus nerve which is being pinched by the HHS. (See Diagram #3.) Whenever the vagus or pelvic nerve is pinched, it produces acid which affects the kidneys. This acid formation, along with poor diet and poor digestion because of the HHS, leads to more acid and improper elimination through the urine and bowels. The more acid there is in the kidney, the higher probability that it will under-function and eventually lead to water retention and the formation of kidney stones.

It is not to say here that kidney imbalances can be quickly alleviated by correcting the HHS, or that kidney stones will instantly dissolve when the stomach is pulled down. What I am stating is that if the stomach is up (HHS), then digestive and nerve disturbances may play a significant part in kidney problems. If you have kidney problems, be sure your stomach is down!

NUTRITIONAL SUGGESTIONS FOR KIDNEY IMBALANCES

1. Always make sure, as well as you're able, that the stomach is down! (Refer to the chapter: "What Can Be Done?")
2. Use natural digestive aids, such as H.H.S. Formula, Pan-Gest or some type of betaine hydrochloride formula. Use the diet outlined in Chapter 34.
3. Drink ½ teaspoon of lemon juice in all water.
4. Drink pure cranberry juice.
5. Make a tea consisting of equal parts of juniper berries, corn silk, and watermelon seeds. Drink 2 times daily.
6. Take juniper berry capsules -- 6 a day.
7. Take buchu leaf capsules -- 6 a day.
8. Fennel Seed Caps -- 1 cap., 3x a day.
9. Flow-Thru, 6 a day. (see mini-catalog)
10. Aspara-Can, 6 a day. (see mini-catalog)

Chapter 10

HEADACHE IMBALANCES

In most cases a headache is the body's wonderful way of signaling that something somewhere else in the system is malfunctioning. In other words, it, too, is a symptom. It is difficult to point a finger at any one thing and say: "That's it! That's what caused my headache!"

The Hiatal Hernia Syndrome (HHS) could be a major factor. It needs to be ruled out by differential diagnosis before dismissing HHS involvement. How might a headache develop as a result of the HHS? First, the stomach goes up. This pinches the vagus nerve and starts a reduction in the amount of hydrochloric acid (HCL) produced; digestion of food is greatly reduced. This brings about a situation of low blood sugar. (See Chapter: "Hypoglycemia".) It is an established fact that low blood sugar leads to headaches, because it reduces the amount of glucose (energy) in the muscles. This causes the neck bones to move out of proper alignment and pinch the nerves in the neck, resulting in further headaches. The cloudiness in thinking that sometimes accompanies headaches comes from the low blood sugar condition. However, the HHS can complicate this type of mental confusion. (See the chapter: "Mental Distress Imbalances".)

Another possibility presents itself when we look at the paths of the stomach and gall bladder meridians in Chinese Medicine. These flow over the head and around the front of the face. If vagus nerve function is disrupted, it can dump excess energy into these pathways or reduce the energy flowing into these paths, thereby causing pain in the head.

Miss E. came in with a "very bad headache, nauseated, dizzy, tired, and a stupid thick feeling in my head," as she worded it. Once the HHS was corrected, she immediately perked up. Most symptoms disappeared with the exception of dizziness and fatigue. These were helped by giving her something to eat to control the low blood sugar symptoms.

Scars and adhesions in the small intestine produce a

reflex action throughout the nervous system, creating muscle spasms in certain areas that misalign the bones and pinch the nerves. The result is most certainly a headache. This, too, can be traced to the HHS (the mother problem) because the vagus nerve causes the small intestine to start under-functioning. Also, the large intestine can become full of toxic waste which toxifies the blood stream, excites the nerves, and causes spinal misalignment in the neck and consequently, headaches.

The migraine headache is somewhat different from the "regular" headache. As with the regular type, I find that in most cases many symptoms of low blood sugar are also present. In addition, clinical experience shows in most cases this crippling pain also stems from digestive disorders and poor hydrochloric acid production. Migraine distress starts with disorientation, sometimes nausea, flashing lights and a type of blind spot in the visual field. The final pain usually settles on one side, many times behind the eyes.

These, too, can be helped by HHS correction. Generally, migraine pain does not diminish as quickly, but I have seen it happen. It takes a while for the energies to settle out with a migraine. Over the long-term, I have found that migraine pain can definitely be alleviated by HHS rebalancing.

Furthermore, I have never found a classical migraine in progress that did not have the HHS. This does not mean that the HHS was the only cause of the migraine, but it is certainly involved.

Brain tumors, genetic brain syndromes, and accidents of the head are not helped by HHS correction. These are totally different situations and require a great deal of medical expertise.

A case in point: Mr. C. came to my office with a migraine that started with flashing lights and blind spots. I found several misalignments occurring at one time and corrected these, but the significant factor was the presence of the HHS. When the stomach was pulled down and he was placed at approximately a 45-degree angle, head up, the pain from the migraine stopped. As long as he stayed at this angle, all was well.

Often migraine sufferers are told that once a migraine is in progress it cannot be stopped until it runs its course. This is not always true in the cases I see, as I stated before. The body never has the intention of staying in such a painful, debilitating state! In many cases, the head has a pressure valve, and if the pressure is eased at the source of disturbance, this takes the pressure off the head and relieves the headache.

Employing logic: If the digestive, nervous, and endocrine systems are at a stage of imbalance, where do these misdirected energies go? The most obvious is back into the head, because it is the origin of body organization. Also, the many bones of the skull are always slightly moving, therefore, enabling pressures to be released. In Holographic Health, our practitioners know how to rebalance these areas and eliminate the pain in a short period.

The next time you suffer a headache, consider the "insidious link." Are you having any of the other HHS symptoms at the same time? Perhaps you have a key in your hand as helpful as aspirin and less harmful to your stomach lining!

NUTRITIONAL SUGGESTIONS FOR HEADACHE IMBALANCES

1. Always make sure, as well as you know how, that the stomach is down! (Refer to chapter: "What Can Be Done?")
2. Use natural digestive aids, such as H.H.S. Formula, Pan-Gest or some type of betaine hydrochloride formula. Use the diet outlined in Chapter 34.
3. In-Sync -- 6 to 12 a day or until the headache is under control and then reduce to 2 a day for maintenance.
4. Feverfew -- 6 a day as needed.
5. White Willow bark capsules - 3 a day as needed.
6. Cherry-Gold -- 6 a day for maintenance; up to 15 a day if migraine is active.
7. Aspara-Can -- 6 a day for maintenance.

Chapter 11

ADRENAL GLAND IMBALANCES

I feel a pressing need to discuss the most immediately affected members of the energy system who suffer from the Hiatal Hernia Syndrome (HHS). These unsung heroes are the adrenal glands. These hard-working little glands are responsible for taking the brunt of negative stresses, poor diet, and many excesses in every facet of our lives.

In my opinion, about two-thirds of the population has under-functioning adrenal glands. It is termed "adrenal sluggishness." An area in the brain called the hypothalamus receives stress signals that stimulate hormones in the hypothalamus called "corticotrophin releasing factor" (CRF). CRF targets in two different directions: first, to the pituitary, causing another hormone, called ACTH, to go to the adrenal glands

Diagram #8A

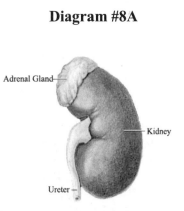

and release cortisol. Cortisol then increases blood sugar and speeds the body's metabolism. Second, it proceeds directly to the adrenal glands. This releases epinephrine which fuels the muscles and brain with extra glucose (energy). Further, the adrenals release norepinephrine, which speeds up the heartbeat and raises the blood pressure. This whole process then loops back to the pituitary, which regulates the stress response further, and causes the adrenal stimulation all over again.

What all this means to you is that moment by moment, day by day, the adrenal glands are forced to overproduce because of our high-stress times. These highly sensitive glands finally just get overused, under-rested and, in many cases, undernourished for so long that they become taxed and energy reserves start decreasing.

What is so interesting to me is that often as soon as the stomach goes up, adrenal sluggishness starts. It is not unusual to watch the adrenal (energy) glands return to normal when the stomach returns to its proper place. If you tax your system again and again, thereby weakening these precious reserves of energy, and the HHS occurs, the adrenal glands can become sluggish no matter what the condition of the stomach. This definitely breeds trouble, and down the primrose path you go - low energy, illness, inability to cope with the day's challenges all become major problems in themselves.

Diagram #8B

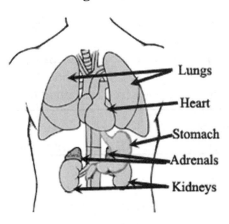

Lungs
Heart
Stomach
Adrenals
Kidneys

An example is Mrs. J. who came in feeling "very fatigued." I found her adrenal glands sluggish. I also found the HHS. After I rebalanced the HHS, she immediately started feeling better. I rechecked the adrenal glands by kinesiology and found they had returned to full strength.

I can unequivocally state that most of the health problems today, having been started by stress, follow this pathway to low adrenals and the HHS. This leads to the specific body area in the individual that is weak. Illness is inevitable.

What I'm giving you in this book is a way out! The stomach is the hub. Something constructive can be done about it. There is hope. At least, you can control the HHS rather than its controlling you!

NUTRITIONAL SUGGESTIONS FOR ADRENAL GLAND IMBALANCES

1. Always make sure, as well as you know how, that the stomach is down! (Refer to the chapter: "What Can Be Done?")
2. Use natural digestive aids, such as H.H.S. Formula, Pan-Gest or some type of betaine hydrochloride formula.
3. Use the diet outlined in Chapter 34.

DAILY

1. Exercise
2. Vitamin A-- 25,000 mg. (Beta carotene)
3. B-Complex
4. Vitamin C -- 2,000 to 7,000 mg.
5. Bee Pollen -- 2 teaspoons a day
6. Ginseng
7. GH3 -- Gerovital
8. Fresh fruits, vegetables, seeds, nuts and grains
9. Reduce red meat, eliminate sugar, and white flour products.
10. Feel Good (an adrenal supplement) -- up to 6 a day
11. Homeopathic adrenal drops - 30 a day for maintenance, up to 60 a day for severe fatigue.
12. Pantothenic acid -- 500 mg., 3x a day
13. Licorice Root -- 500 mg., 3x a day
14. Cayenne -- 500 mg., 3x a day
15. Have quiet periods of prayer and meditation.

Chapter 12

HEART IMBALANCES

"Surely you don't expect me to believe that a hiatal hernia is linked to heart problems," Mr C. said.

"More than that, Mr. C.," I replied. "The HHS often leads to what is called a pseudo-heart attack. You think for sure you are having an actual one. There is even pain down the left arm, occasionally accompanied by intense chest pain, rapid heart beat and profuse sweating. Believe it or not, this could be just another symptom of the insidious link, the Hiatal Hernia Syndrome."

Mr. C. was silent for a moment, pondering these new thoughts. Finally he said, "So that's what happened to me. I thought I was a goner for sure."

"Well, Mr. C., I hear this relatively often in my office. In fact, I think that the Hiatal Hernia Syndrome could lead to true heart attacks. It can happen this way. Once the stomach goes up, there is a reduction in digestive ability. This means that the body cannot turn its food into usable nutrients and energy for the cells. Slowly, it starves. Because of improper digestion the body will store the food you eat in the fat cells, so you gain weight and still feel weak. This can be the beginning of low blood sugar problems. (See Chapter: "Hypoglycemia".) Then, your endocrine system becomes sluggish. A reduction of adrenal and thyroid production can then cause the beginning of the heart problem. Also, the increased fatty deposits collect around the organs. There is an elevation of cholesterol and triglycerides in the blood. Both these put more of a strain on the heart. Furthermore, there seems to be a reflex action from the vagus nerve where it is pinched when the stomach goes up, for this nerve also has very important branches going into the heart and could interfere with heart function. Add all of this, counting the fact that your heart is crowded by the stomach, and you see how the HHS and heart problems can be linked."
Mr. C., having been patient and pensive for awhile, then said: "Why don't my other doctors know about this?" I replied,

"Perhaps your own story will help them to understand."

Many people, as Mr. C., are questioning and looking in all directions for help with heart disease. Whatever your persuasion, be it layperson or professional - if you see this problem in your family or neighbor, show him this book. Let him know there may be something more: -- an "insidious link."

NUTRITIONAL SUGGESTIONS FOR HEART IMBALANCES

1. Always make sure, as well as you know how, that the stomach is down! (Refer to Chapter: "What Can Be Done?"')
2. Use natural digestive aids, such as H.H.S. Formula, Pan-Gest or some type of betaine hydrochloride formula.
3. Use the diet outlined in Chapter 34.

DAILY

1. B-Complex or B-Well or Bee Powerful -- 2 a day
2. Vitamin C (1000 mg) -- 3x a day or Complete C -- 2 a day
3. Vitamin. E -- 100 IU, increasing 100 IU per week until 1000 IU is reached.
4. Lecithin
5. Kelp -- three tablets a day
6. Sociable garlic -- two to three capsules a day
7. Alpha-Omega (essential fatty acids) -- 1 to 2 a day
8. Selenium
9. Calcium and magnesium supplements or Magnesium Penetrator 1 to 2 in the morning and Calcium Penetrator -- 2 to 4 at bedtime.
10. Cod liver oil
11. Potassium -- to be used if diuretics are being taken.
12. Kleen Sweep -- an oral chelating substance, also good for the removal of chemicals and heavy metals - Start with 3 a day and go up to 6 over 2 months.
13. Heart-Line -- 3 to 6 a day
14. Blood Harmonizer -- at least 3 a day if you have high cholesterol.

Avoid all stimulants! (e.g. coffee, tea, tobacco, sugar, salt, alcohol, red meat, soft drinks, white bread or any processed foods.)

Chapter 13

CHOLESTEROL IMBALANCES

The reason doctors pay so much attention to cholesterol is that it appears to be one of the main indicators of the condition of arteries and possible heart involvement. It is not the only major culprit, as many people believe. There are some authorities who now think that it seems to have little to do with the overall problem. Some feel that triglycerides are the real problem and others that certain fractions of the LDL (Low Density Lipids) and HDL (High Density Lipids) are all that matter. A good friend who is in the medical field told me that he had a patient whose cholesterol, triglyceride, EKG and blood pressure numbers were all perfect and died the afternoon after the tests of a massive heart attack at forty-three.

Are the Hiatal Hernia Syndrome (HHS) and cholesterol connected? Again, I contend that the HHS causes faulty digestion and assimilation.

Just what is cholesterol? What does it do? It is a substance produced in the liver (about 2 grams a day.) Cholesterol is necessary for the production of the sex hormones, adrenal (energy) hormones, bile salts, and the transport of essential fatty acids. It is also a constituent of the skin, a covering of nerve fibers, and is essential to the normal functioning of the immune system, particularly the body's response to such invaders as cancer cells. Our bodies simply could not function without it.

Then' why does it reach dangerously high levels in our blood? Is it our diet? Well, partly so, but more importantly, the reason lies in what we digest and assimilate. I have seen the most careful of eaters with low cholesterol diets who have a high level in the blood. Cholesterol also has a cohort -- triglycerides. Often, when triglyceride levels are high, so are cholesterol levels and vice versa.

If the process of digestion is so crucial to the proper utilization of cholesterol and triglycerides, then what happens if digestion is impaired? As always this leads us back to the presence of the HHS, the very culprit that points to poor assimilation of food.

Now, let's go one step further. Digestion affects the function of the adrenal glands, and they become sluggish. Remember that cholesterol helped to make up certain adrenal hormones? We now have extra cholesterol that should be used for our energy glands but remains unused. Also, remember that cholesterol is necessary for the production of bile salts in the liver. What happens if the liver is sluggish, too? In many cases, I see this faulty function in the liver cells which sends added cholesterol into the blood because the liver can't utilize it to produce bile salts. This, in turn, affects digestion even further by bile salt reduction!

Where does *that* leave us? In short, it leaves us with a high amount of cholesterol in the blood. Cholesterol is so important; we have to look at it as having money (cholesterol) in the bank (bloodstream) but no checkbook to get it out. I have seen definite clinical results that indicate the use of adrenal gland and blood balancing nutritional supplements in sufficient amounts can reduce blood cholesterol levels. There is sound reasoning for this. Physiology shows us that high triglycerides are decreased by adrenal hormones and the elimination of sugar from the diet. This means that cholesterol is also decreased by additional adrenal support.

Correct the HHS first! Allow proper digestion and assimilation of your food to occur.

NUTRITIONAL SUGGESTIONS TO REDUCE CHOLESTEROL IMBALANCES

For cholesterol to be made and utilized, adrenal hormones must be in sufficient amounts as well as something to energetically and nutritionally stabilize the blood.

1. Always make sure, as well as you can, that the stomach is down! (Refer to Chap 34: "What Can Be Done?")
2. Use natural digestive aids, such as H.H.S. Formula, Pan-Gest or some type of betaine hydrochloride formula.
3. Use the diet outlined in Chapter 34.

DAILY

It is recommended to avoid red meat, processed and refined food, tobacco, caffeine, tea and alcohol.

1. Feel Good (an adrenal supplement) -- 6 daily

2. Blood Harmonizer -- 4 to 6 daily
3. Complete C -- 4 a day
4. Zinc Penetrator -- 1 a day
5. Vitamin E -- up to 800 IU daily
6. Phosphytidal Choline -- 2 gel caps a day
7. Cayenne pepper capsules
8. Kleen Sweep -- 3 a day

Chapter 14

OBESITY IMBALANCES

I weep when I approach this highly misunderstood topic, for this condition afflicts more than the body of its sufferers. It affects their image of themselves. They will undertake any endeavor to lose weight. The desperation that I hear in the voices of those that walk in my office is disheartening.

I do not promise weight loss; this is not my nutritional focus. I am devoted to returning the body to a high state of integrated balance. Since it is the glands that determine body metabolism and weight, rebalancing the HHS can be supportive to weight loss efforts.

The integration of glandular function is often devastated when the HHS is in progress. How can the precious body be expected to function adequately when the food entering it cannot be assimilated and feed the glands that regulate its balance?

Excess weight is also held in the body by poisons and other tissue acid wastes. They hold water and fat in the cells and in-between the cells. To enhance weight loss metabolism, reduce these poison by-products caused by HHS disruption.

In my opinion, this is what happens after the HHS involves itself to create obesity:

1. Because of lowered hydrochloric acid in the stomach which fails to break down food at the proper body rate, a person does not get the nutrition from his food exactly when it is needed. This creates a desire for more food soon after a meal. If more food is then eaten, even though it is in excess, the body stores this in the fat tissue as available energy to be used when called for by the system. It takes a great deal more food ingested, and more frequently, to provide the body with its basic nutritional requirements.

2. Food not properly digested becomes poisonous acid waste products. These waste products lower the adrenal gland's ability to function, and puts a burden on

the thyroid gland to maintain correct energy reserves. This directly affects blood sugar balance in the body. The adrenal glands begin to under-function. As a result, these adrenal hormones that would have contributed to bringing stored fat back into energy usage are not available to do so. Thus, another helper to dissolve utilizable fat is diminished.

3.   A low functioning thyroid is almost always a factor in obesity, perhaps as a result of diminished adrenal function. Thyroxin (the thyroid hormone) acts like soap and dissolves fat. In any case, low thyroid action is a major contributor to obesity.

A simple test that you can do to check your own thyroid level is given at the end of this chapter.

There are many reasons for obesity and I am touching only on a few. The pituitary gland and hypothalamus area of the brain may be malfunctioning. Psychological factors could play a very prominent part because of a lowered self image. I have seen enough evidence in my own practice to make me believe that too often the HHS is a primary factor overlooked in obesity also.

Make sure the stomach is down first. This should make your attempts at weight loss more productive.

HYPOTHYROID TEST

Each morning before getting out of bed, place an oral thermometer underneath your arm pit. Leave it there for 10 minutes. Record the temperature. Do this for 5 days (For ladies, do not begin this testing on the first day of your menstrual cycle.)

To evaluate this test, 97.8 degrees is low normal. 98.2 degrees is high normal. Anything below 97.8 degrees suggests a low thyroid profile. Check with your holistic physician if you show a subnormal reading.

NUTRITIONAL SUGGESTIONS FOR OBESITY

1.   Always make sure, as well as you're able, that the stomach is down! (Refer to Chapter: "What Can Be Done?")
2.   Use natural digestive aids, such as H.H.S. Formula, Pan-Gest or some type of betaine hydrochloride formula.

3.　There are as many food diets as there are people when it comes to losing weight. Here is a brief synopsis of my program:

- **To increase digestive ability, make sure the HHS is rebalanced.**
- **To reduce the accumulation of any toxins which interfere with assimilation of food nutrients, creating a state of chronic hunger.**
- **To eliminate poisons.**

(More is explained in our free catalog. Call us for a copy.)

4.　This is done by increasing the fiber in your diet, the breathing exercises, drinking enough water, and certain nutrients in the formulas listed next that work very mildly.

5.　Take 2 Trim-Silver at bedtime. If you feel you can handle more after 3 days, go to 3 at bedtime. Wait another week and if you feel you can tolerate more, go to 4 at bedtime.

6.　Take 1 of the 12 Systems Synergistic Multiples with each meal.

7.　Take 1 to 2 of the Extreme Greens with each meal.

8.　Take 2 Can-Clear at bedtime if you are not having at least one very good bowel movement a day.

9.　Ask about our Trim-It-Up program.

10.　I would suggest a book by Dr. Ann Wigmore entitled From <u>Fat to Fit</u> as another alternative to approaching this imbalance.

11.　Let your nutritionally-minded health professional help you determine if you need any natural hormonal support. Often the adrenal, thyroid, pituitary, and/or hypothalamus can be energetically weakened in obesity.

12.　Reduce your carbohydrate intake to no more than 40 grams a day; less is even better. (Supervision is suggested). Many people are allergic to carbohydrates. Get yourself a carbohydrate counter booklet at your health food store.

Chapter 15

HYPOGLYCEMIA IMBALANCES
(LOW BLOOD SUGAR)

The absence of digestive enzymes and hydrochloric acid production leads to unhealthy bodies. I start to suspect many interrelated syndromes at this point. I am estimating that approximately 85% of the overall populace has the affliction of the Hiatal Hernia Syndrome (HHS).

Over the last 10 years, biochemically nutrition-minded physicians of every discipline have noted a very high number of functional low blood sugar cases. In my experience and the experience of other colleagues, it has been observed that the Glucose Tolerance Test for low blood sugar does not always provide a positive diagnosis, even after 5 hours or more. Yet, the patient will continually have every characteristic symptom of low blood sugar. The customary holistic practice is to proceed with a corrective diet and watch for results. Usually, if digestive ability is restored, moderate to excellent results occur in a short period of time.

It intrigues me that part of low blood sugar symptomology, which includes fatigue, low energy, listlessness, and irritability, is the exact same things I find in people with the HHS. In my opinion, the HHS is the mother of this condition too.

In hypoglycemia, we must look at the stomach first. What can be expected if the stomach is not assimilating food? The body operates on a substance called <u>glucose.</u> Glucose is the "gasoline" to run our vehicle. It is made by the food we eat and *assimilate*. In other words, it is the crude oil from which the refinery produces gasoline as an end product. The gasoline (glucose) is put into the gas tank (blood) and runs along the gas lines (circulatory system) to the engine. Our main engine (glucose user) in the body is the brain. When blood sugar (glucose) drops, the first area affected is the brain. This causes disorientation, inability to focus attention fully, and even a failing memory in many cases.

A low blood sugar syndrome (hypoglycemia) allows the entire body to run down rather quickly. I have seen people who cannot stay awake, who sleep most of the time, and even hide themselves away in depression. Carl Pfeiffer, M.D., who worked with numerous cases of mental distress, reported low blood sugar symptoms in many of them.

How does this tie into the HHS? Rather nicely. What happens is this. There is an interference with hydrochloric acid production and digestive enzyme production when the stomach goes up, which starts the process of low blood sugar (hypoglycemia). The hypoglycemic condition then creates all the above symptoms.

Is the first step in low blood sugar then a result of HHS? Is this why we have equal percentages of people (85%) with the HHS and (85%) that have hypoglycemia?

NUTRITIONAL SUGGESTIONS FOR HYPOGLYCEMIA IMBALANCES
Always make sure, as well as you're able, that the stomach is down! (Refer to Chap 34: "What Can Be Done?") Avoid all refined foods, sugars, white flours, soft drinks.
1. Use natural digestive aids, such as H.H.S. Formula, Pan-Gest or some type of betaine hydrochloride formula.
2. Use the diet outlined in Chapter 34.

DAILY
1. Take a good multi-vitamin formula with minerals, herbs, and enzymes, such as 12-System Synergistic Multiple at 3X a day.
2. A super B-complex such as Bee Powerful or a liquid such as B-Well -- 2x a day.
3. Vitamin C--2000 to 5000 mg. a day or Complete C -- 4 a day.
4. Feel Good or some type of raw adrenal food supplement at least 3X a day. (Do not take at supper.)
5. Spirulina -- 3 a day, or 2 tablespoons of powder/day.
6. Protein powder -- 3x a day.
7. Liquid trace minerals (There are several different companies that have these) -- 10 drops, 3x a day.
8. Fennel Seed Caps -- 1 cap., 3x a day.

Chapter 16

ALCOHOLISM IMBALANCES

It is said of alcoholism: "Being an alcoholic is the deepest darkest, most hopeless place one can look from." Can the Hiatal Hernia Syndrome (HHS) be related to alcoholism? Yes, the "insidious link" wraps its tendrils around yet another phase of illness.

It is well known that low blood sugar (hypoglycemia) and high blood sugar (diabetes) often accompany alcoholism. Look at the symptoms that low blood sugar brings and see its patterns - fatigue, depression, loss of hope. Add a few serious emotional and financial problems, and it is easy to understand how one would be led to drink.

Alcohol provides no beneficial nutrition to the body, and by hardening the liver it can cause digestive enzymes to function poorly. Add to this, vagus nerve stimulation when large portions of alcohol enter the body, particularly without solid food to accompany it. The vagus nerve causes the stomach to over secrete hydrochloric acid, and this produces a contraction and spasm in the stomach and diaphragm. Subsequently, the stomach is pulled up, and problems with the HHS start. This makes the low blood sugar worse. Concurrently, alcohol has a very negative effect on the function of the adrenal glands, which provide our energy and help to regulate proper levels of blood sugar.

One of the problems always found in alcoholism is high triglyceride and cholesterol levels. If the adrenal glands were working properly, these levels would be kept in balance. (See Chapter: "Cholesterol Imbalances".)

Will the HHS correction cure alcoholism? It certainly will not. Every alcoholic I have had the chance to examine had an HHS. I think this is more than coincidence. The least that can be done to help those in this nutritionally starving situation is to correct the digestion as much as possible. Then, they may have a chance to get above their depression. The link to what is happening with the blood sugar levels of an alcoholic and what the HHS does to promote low blood sugar and adrenal insufficiency should not be denied. The best way to start with the correction of digestion is to start with the realignment of the Hiatal Hernia Syndrome.

NUTRITIONAL SUGGESTIONS FOR ALCOHOLISM

Excessive drinking creates a vicious cycle by depleting the body of vitamins, especially severe deficiencies in B-complex vitamins. Alcohol causes damage to the brain, pancreas, duodenum, and liver as well as causing a definite depression of the auto-immune system.

1. Always make sure, as well as you're able, that the stomach is down! (Refer to Chapter: "What Can Be Done?")
2. Use natural digestive aids, such as H.H.S. Formula, Pan-Gest or some type of betaine hydrochloride formula.
3. Use the diet outlined in Chapter 34.

DAILY

1. Vitamin A -- 25,000 IU (Beta carotene).
2. B-complex 6 tablets, 3x a day -- or Bee Powerful 3 daily.
3. B-6 -- 10 mg.
4. Vitamin C -- 3000 mg or Complete C -- 6 daily.
5. Vitamin D -- 400IU.
6. Vitamin E -- up to 1000IU.
7. Zinc Orotate or Picolinate -- 60 mg. or Zinc Penetrator -- 2 a day.
8. 12 Systems Synergistic Multiple -- 3 a day.
9. Butcher's Broom -- 1 capsule, 3x a day.
10. Raw adrenal in combination with herbs and thymus tissue (or use Feel Good- - 6 a day). This could be a whole therapy in itself for alcoholism. Depending upon the severity of the condition, I would recommend 10 tablets a day of at least 80 mg. per tablet, taken at a rate of two tablets, 5x a day, plus the need for homeopathic adrenal, several times a day. These can be found in most of health stores.
11. Fresh fruits and vegetables.

Chapter 17

FOOD AND ENVIRONMENTAL
SENSITIVITIES/ ALLERGEN IMBALANCES

The connection between food/environmental sensitivities and allergies and the Hiatal Hernia Syndrome (HHS) is one of profound significance to those millions of people who suffer these reactions. The role of digestion and proper assimilation is often ignored by health care practitioners who see patients with these problems. What needs to be examined here is not the established fact of food or environmental allergies, but what causes you, the sufferer, to have to endure them.

One of the basic facts about our marvelous bodies is that we have a defense system already built into it -- the auto-immune system. It has various branches, but the central gland that runs the job of body self-defense is the thymus gland. (See Diagram #9.) This wonderful gland was, until 1953, thought to be useless. Present day research is proving different.

The thymus gland produces what is called lymphocytes (T-cells and B-cells) and sends these infection fighters to the scene of any battle for survival. It does this through its network, which it supplies and keeps stimulated to produce more infection-fighters. These other members of the defense team are the lymph nodes and the spleen. To

Diagram #9

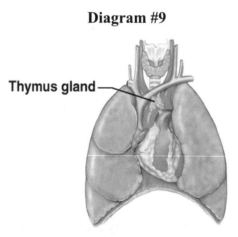

Thymus gland

give you an idea about the size and importance of the lymph system, it is just as extensive as our circulatory system and is always on guard.

When there is an allergy attack, the body should produce its own antihistamines. An acute reaction results

72

when the body produces too few of them because there is an imbalance in the adrenal glands. The adrenal glands can malfunction over a period of months or years causing the energy level of the body to decrease. Sometimes this decrease is dramatic. This in turn affects the autoimmune system.

The allergy sufferer gets caught in the crossfire.
1. The adrenal glands that supply natural antihistamine action to protect you become sluggish.
2. This sluggishness and lowering of energy leads to the lowering of thymus function, which leaves you wide open for adverse reactions from anything - whether it be food or inhalants.

To put it another way: because of biochemical imbalances and glandular sluggishness, you become a sitting duck. Your enemies multiply, as your immune system's inadequacies increase. Today, it is corn to which you are allergic. Tomorrow, it is dust. Tuesday, it is wheat, and so on.

Now, enter the dragon, the un-thought-of, the "mother of all illness," the HHS. I have observed some very interesting connections between the immune system, the adrenal glands and allergies.

Most people I examine a person with moderate to severe allergies show an HHS! At first, I was quite surprised by this and questioned myself constantly. Further investigation made things clearer. As always when the HHS occurs, there is a definite disturbance of hydrochloric acid production and digestive enzymes which are responsible for breaking down foods and making them usable. If your digestion and assimilation are disrupted, the body will eventually have blood sugar problems. (See the Chapter "Hypoglycemia Imbalances".) When the body does not get what it needs, glands are strained and weakened. The adrenal glands seem particularly susceptible to stress and malnutrition. This takes us to the next logical step of thymus gland and immune system sluggishness. From here it is possible to see how allergies could occur as a result of these body defense breakdowns.

To Summarize:
1. The HHS causes a problem with improper assimilation of nutrients, therefore causing a malnourished and

weakened system.

2. When under attack, the adrenal glands become sluggish and no longer produce adequate amounts of antihistamines in the system.
3. The thymus gland and auto-immune system reduce proper body defense.
4. This leaves the person susceptible (allergic) to certain foods and inhalants he might easily have handled before.

A case in point: Mrs. M. came to me. She had severely crippling allergic reactions to a great number of foods, as well as to plants and inhalants of all kinds. I found the HHS and corrected it. With the addition of hydrochloric acid supplementation, she began to feel stronger and look better. Soon her previous allergy problems with foods began to lessen and even disappear. Yet every time there was a recurrence, I found the need to treat the HHS.

Another interesting case is A.C. She has had a chronic problem with devastating headaches caused by large numbers of allergies. I found the HHS. Her headaches stop immediately and her energy level is quickly restored with the correction of the HHS. What's the connection between these allergies and her headaches? Undoubtedly, it is through the "insidious link," the HHS, and the way it affects her particular situation with allergy.

I am not saying that the HHS causes allergies. I am saying that it is the "mother problem" in many cases which provides the physiological breakdowns that set up allergic reactions.

NUTRITIONAL SUGGESTIONS FOR FOOD AND ENVIRONMENTAL SENSITIVITIES/ALLERGENS IMBALANCES

These can apply to asthma, sinus trouble, headaches, and colon problems. I would suggest allergy testing done by Immuno Laboratories, Inc. Let your health practitioner help you with this. This lab is excellent for foods and environmental imbalances. Other allergy testing procedures may be helpful, but I find this one to be reliable.

1. Always make sure, as well as you know how, that the stomach is down! (Refer to Chapter: "What Can Be Done?")

74

2. Use natural digestive aids, such as H.H.S. Formula, Pan-Gest or some type of betaine hydrochloride formula.
3. Use the diet outlined in Chapter 34.
4. Rotate your foods, so that you will eat only each item four days apart. Example: Eat potatoes on Monday and Friday only.

DAILY

1. A vitamin C supplement such as Complete C - up to 10 a day or 5000 mgs. of a vitamin C powder according to the seriousness of the reaction.
2. Free Breath -- 6 to 9 a day (helps all types of allergies, asthma and lung disorders.)
3. B-complex -- 50 - 100 mg. or Bee Powerful -- 3 a day or B-Well liquid, 2 tsps. daily
4. Vitamin A -- 25,000 IU beta carotene
5. Vitamin D -- 400 1U.
6. Vitamin E -- up to 800 IU. Start with 100 IU and increase to 100 IU every three days until reaching 800 IU.
7. Calcium Penetrator -- up to 2 at bedtime.
8. Pantothenic acid -- 100 mg. or up to 200 mg. Do not exceed this amount without a doctor's supervision. However, larger doses are helpful. It is my opinion that this is true because of pantothenic acid's support of the adrenal glands.
9. Bee pollen --- One-half teaspoon a day.
10. Raw adrenal tablets -- 4x a day at least 100 mg. each. or Feel Good -- 3+ a day.
11. Potassium Penetrator -- 1 a day.
12. Butcher's Broom -- 1 capsule, 3x a day.
13. Raw Thymus extract -- 2 tablets, 3x a day or Infect Away-- 6 a day. (Immune system support)
14. Fennel Seed Caps -- 1 cap.-3x a day.
15. Flush Out --- a great sinus bath. Stops infections.
16. No smoking.

Avoid caffeine, chocolate, eggs, tomatoes, wheat, dairy products, oysters, salmon, refined foods, food colorings. This is not a complete list by any means, and these foods should be challenged to be determined if they are indeed culprits by some sort of testing procedure.

Chapter 18

STRESS IMBALANCES

We are all victims of the stresses of everyday life. There is also a very negative love affair secretly going on as a result of this stress. It exists between our delicate stomach and a ruthless self-imposing dictator. That dictator is *internalized stress.*

The diaphragm is the breathing muscle. When the stomach goes up too far out of its normal position, the Hiatal Hernia Syndrome (HHS) is the result. Stress causes the ascending of the stomach through the diaphragm. The stomach area is so tender and incredibly sensitive that the way you treat every aspect of yourself (physical, emotional, mental and spiritual) will in some way show up in your stomach area. Understanding the relationship between stress and the HHS is important because, without realizing it, you may be perpetuating the problem, perhaps even minute by minute.

There is logic for this. The stomach and the second largest number of nerve interconnections in the body, called the solar plexus, are in the same place. So important is this zone of nerves that it has been called our "second brain." There is direct effect upon the stomach if the function of this area is disrupted in any way. Becoming frustrated, upset, or angry causes tension in this area; the vagus nerve stimulates the body to secrete large amounts of hydrochloric acid when it is not necessary; then there is contraction in the stomach and a spasm in the diaphragm which leads to the HHS and its multitude of symptoms.

There is more to it than this. Stress is actually learned! When taxing situations occur, we habitually perceive and deal with them in certain ways. If we don't cope well, then the stomach tightens. Energy increases at first, but it will be a scattered type of energy and lasts only as long as the particular nervous system tolerates it. Indeed, some people don't last long these days because of the rapid pace. It extends the energy systems to the limit. Day after day as the stomach, tightens the cycle is repeated. Finally, a small tear may occur in the diaphragm. In time this tear may enlarge and push the stomach through the small opening. The HHS with all its dark implications begins. (See Diagram #5.)

In his book, *Psychological Stress and the Coping Process,* Richard Lazarus states the causes of stress:
1. You are in a situation where some demand or stressor exits.
2. You recognize and evaluate the demand and then realize you can't cope with it.
3. You respond inadequately.
4. Negative consequences follow.

I deduce that the nervous system learns helplessness from this inadequate response. The feeling of helplessness inundates all other areas in us. The stomach area unremittingly tightens, as we continue to respond inadequately and the HHS thrives.

Stress can also be viewed in relation to the HHS as an imbalance between demands in day-to-day living and our capability to cope with them. These events are further described in the **Social Readjustment Rating Scale** constructed by Holmes and Rahe using Life Change Units (LCU). They state that if you score 300 points you have an 80% chance of getting sick in the near future. From 150-299 points you have a 50% chance. Less than 150 points and you will have about a 30% chance.

Rate yourself on this scale to find your stress level; then apply the score in the next scale.

SOCIAL READJUSTMENT RATING SCALE

Rank Life Event	Mean Value
Death of spouse	100
Divorce	73
Marital separation	65
Jail term	63
Death of close family member	63
Personal injury or illness	53
Marriage	50

Rank Life Event	Mean Value
Fired at work	47
Marital reconciliation	45
Retirement	45
Change in health of family member	44
Pregnancy	40
Sex difficulties	39
Gain of new family member	39
Business readjustment	39
Change in financial state	38
Death of close friend	37
Change to different line of work	36
Change in # of arguments with spouse	35
Mortgage over $10,000	31
Foreclosure of mortgage of loan	30
Change in responsibilities at work	29
Son or daughter leaving home	29
Trouble with in-laws	29
Outstanding personal achievements	28
Wife begin or stop work	26
Begin or end school	26
Change in living conditions	25
Revision of personal habits	24
Trouble with boss	23
Change in work hours or conditions	20
Change in residence	20
Change in schools	20
Change in recreation	19
Change in church activities	19
Change in social activities	18
Mortgage or loan less than $10,000	17
Change in sleeping habits	16
Change in number of family get-togethers	15
Change in eating habits	15
Vacation	13
Christmas	12
Minor violations of the law	11

After seeing hundreds of patients who have the Hiatal Hernia Syndrome, I am certain that at least 85% of our population has the HHS at one time or another. I would evaluate individual probability this way. Using your score from above, rate yourself on this scale:

300 points	HHS 90% of the time
250 - 299 points	HHS 80% of the time
200 - 249 points	HHS 70% of the time
150 - 249 points	HHS 65% of the time
100 - 149 points	HHS 50% of the time
99 - 0 points	HHS in many smaller percentages or not at all.

Not only do certain events produce stress but so do our attitudes:

ATTITUDES

That Create Stress:	That Alleviate Stress:
Fear	Lovingness
Anger	Laughter
Hate	Enthusiasm
Jealousy	Joy
Moodiness	Sense of Humor

To express these attitudes despite stressful situations can greatly benefit our bodies as we go through major life events. My own experience with patients has convinced me that even a minor amount of stress, which could cause the HHS, presents the possibility of starting down the inevitable path to sickness and poor health.

Stress release exercises I have found useful in my practice are illustrated in the chapter, "What You Can Do for Yourself".

NUTRITIONAL SUGGESTIONS FOR STRESS
1. Always make sure, as well as you're able, that the stomach is down! (Refer Chap. 34: "What Can Be Done?")
2. Use natural digestive aids, such as H.H.S. Formula, Pan-Gest or some type of betaine hydrochloride formula.
3. Use the diet outlined in Chapter 34.

DAILY
1. Raw adrenal supplement -- 3 a day or Feel Good 3 a day.
2. Potassium Penetrator -- 1 a day.
3. Bee Powerful -- 3 a day or Brewer's Yeast.
4. Valerian root tea daily at bedtime.

5. B-Complex -- 3 tablets, 3x a day.
6. Vitamin C- - 3000 mg. to 7000 mg. daily.
7. L-lysine-- 100 mg a day (Use this if you have problems with Herpes because excessive stress will definitely brings on an outbreak.) or Back-Off -- 1 to 2 a day. This was specifically made to help with herpes imbalances of all types.
8. Inositol -- 500 mg. - 2x a day.
9. Calcium Penetrator -- 2 to 4 at bedtime.
10. Herbs that are helpful: Skullcap, passion flower, licorice root, cayenne pepper, chamomile, and valerian root.
11. Take Epsom Salts Bath -- 3 cups in hot bath water. Soak 15 minutes; then shower. Do this before bed.

Chapter 19

MENTAL DISTRESS IMBALANCES

The key to understanding mental distress is linked to chemical imbalances. We know that energy levels decrease because of the involvement with low blood sugar when the HHS is in progress. Often a symptom of low blood sugar is moderate to severe depression. Some people are very chemically sensitive, and they manifest this loss of energy and confusion in a violent, disoriented way.

I cannot state that the Hiatal Hernia Syndrome (HHS) causes mental instability. However, I have found indirect connections. To begin with, note that many HHS sufferers experience a lack of mental acuity. This can range from mild confusion to marked confusion of general reasoning abilities.

A case in point, Mrs. H.: After correcting the HHS she reported a greater ability to remain calm and orient her body. The problem dealt with blurred perception for her. It definitely opened up a whole new world because her energy was no longer scattered. Her words to me: "I used to have to move all the time because of the need to orient myself. This no longer occurs after the HHS is corrected. If disorientation occurs again, I know that my stomach is up and you have shown me how to correct it."

Another patient, an accomplished pianist, knows when the stomach is up because he can't perform on the piano as well. He reported better concentration and concert performance after the HHS was corrected.

Another instance is Mrs. C.: When the HHS is up, not only does her energy drop drastically, but her ability to think clearly goes down. She went to several psychologists and psychiatrists, thinking she was "crazy," as she put it. As soon as the HHS was corrected, the change in her energy, her outlook, and her general sense of well being was so different as to be startling.

At first I did not believe such a thing possible, but case after case supports my conviction.

Even more startling to me is the case of Mr. W., diagnosed as a manic-depressive for many years. His almost total dissociation from reality always began with tightness just below the sternum (breast bone), the major diagnostic point for the HHS. He reported that after a couple of days this tightness would expand into his chest and true anxiety would begin. I examined him, found the HHS, and was able to alleviate these symptoms by realigning it.

It is no mystery to me why the ancient Greeks called the area just below the sternum "the hypochondria" meaning, upper abdomen. It has a further and deeper meaning in modern times. A hypochondriac is a person who is constantly restless and generally over-concerned about the state of his health. This is often what I see in relation to this area. With what are we dealing? I feel it is the same thing that the ancient Greeks and other cultures of the past have dealt with -- "the mother of all illness," the HHS.

Another patient, Mrs. J., came in suffering from a deep mood of depression. Astoundingly, she felt better immediately after the HHS correction. "It is as though something deep and dark was just lifted from my chest," she reported.

Undoubtedly, this syndrome plays a part in many serious cases of mental imbalance. More clinical experience needs to be gathered. If the HHS does play even a minor role in more serious long-term chronic disorders, wouldn't it be worth considering? This field of HHS research is essentially brand new. Perhaps someone reading this book will be the one to research and write conclusively about this "insidious link" and all its subtle mental manifestations. The challenge is yours!

NUTRITIONAL SUGGESTIONS FOR MENTAL DISTRESS

1. Always make sure, as well as you know how, that the stomach is down! (Refer to Chapter: "What Can Be Done?")
2. Use natural digestive aids, such as H.H.S. Formula, Pan-Gest or some type of betaine hydrochloride formula.
3. Use the diet outlined in Chapter 34. Be sure you aren't suffering from food allergies or hypoglycemia. Avoid sugar, processed foods, soft drinks, caffeine and white flour.
4. Vitamin C -- 3000 to 5000 mg. or Complete C -- 6 a day.

5. B-Complex -- 4 tablets, 3x a day or B-Well -- 2 teas. daily
6. Butcher's Broom -- 2 capsules, 3x a day
7. L-Glutamine (amino acid) -- 4 teaspoons a day
8. Mood Mender -- 4 to 6 a day
9. Spirulina -- 1 capsule a day
10. GH-3 -- Gerovital
11. Brewer's Yeast
12. Fo-Ti Tieng -- 500 mg., --- 3x a day
13. Gotu-Kola -- 500 mg. - 3x a day
14. Ginseng -- for males 500 mg.-- 2x a day
15. Dong Quai -- for females 500 mg. -- 2x a day
16. Fennel Seed Caps -- 1 cap. --3X a day
17. St.John's Wort Tincture -- 10 drops -- 1X a day
18. L-Tyrosine --4 a day
19. Chestnut powder -- 1 tsp. daily or 2 caps. daily[1]

---

[1] Note: Ginseng and Dong Quai may be taken by either gender. Ginseng seems to work better for the male hormones, and Dong Quai works well with the female hormones.

Chapter 20

BACKACHE IMBALANCES

One of the most interesting aspects of this work is the relationship between the Hiatal Hernia Syndrome (HHS) and spinal pain. I find many areas of spinal pain that are relieved

Diagram #10

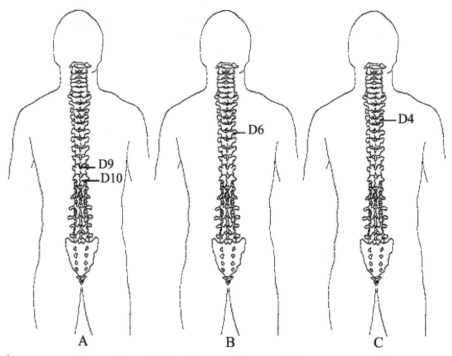

by correcting the HHS disruption. There are, of course, anatomical reasons for this. For example, the relationship between the mid-back areas from the 4th thoracic to the 9th thoracic is evident. (See Diagram #10A, B, C) The manipulation of these areas by qualified licensed professionals can definitely bring relief to some of the symptoms surrounding the HHS, especially if the manipulation at these levels allows the stomach to relax into proper position once again.

A case in point: Mrs. J. came to me with spinal pain from the top of her head to the bottom of her tail bone. She also complained of aches in the various other joints, knees, elbows, hands and feet. I did conservative spinal manipulation and she felt relieved "all over," as she put it. However she came back several times in about a two-week period with exactly the same complaints. Each time she would get complete relief, only to return with the same pains all over again. This concerned me, as I could not understand why she was improving only immediately after a treatment. Several visits later I became suspicious and asked her when the pain recurred. She told me that it came at night while she was in bed. She also said that the spinal pain at that time went from zero to a hundred in severity, and she felt she couldn't breathe. This gave me more reason for suspicion, and I decided to check her for the HHS. I found that there was involvement. Making the simple corrections as are illustrated in the chapter, "What You Can Do For Yourself" the pain in her entire body actually disappeared! This was done *before* I did spinal manipulation!

I found a similar case with Mrs. S. The remarkable thing about both of these was that the only symptom they displayed overtly, besides intense spinal pain, was shortness of breath. Since this symptom had been with them for some time, they both paid little or no attention to it and only acknowledged it upon questioning. This was my first clue that the HHS was in progress. From there I deduced that spinal pain is related in a significant way to the Hiatal Hernia Syndrome.

Pain in and under the left shoulder blade is a rather common complaint. Spinal manipulation helps unless the HHS is in progress. If so, freedom from pain will be temporary or non-existent. Suspicion and logic once again led me to correct the HHS first. To my surprise, the insistent left shoulder pain vanished. A case in point: Mrs. C. had gained relief from a number of chronic spinal problems that she said "hurt a lot all the time," but could not seem to get any consistent relief from her left shoulder pain. After correction of "the mother of all illness" and *before* spinal manipulation, the pain was gone.

There is also the case of Mrs. H., who reported feeling like "a golf ball was always under her left shoulder." She had instant relief after correction of the HHS.

Another case in point: Mrs. M. complained of pain under

the right shoulder, and I found the HHS. Subsequent correction stopped this pain instantly.

It is interesting to me how elusive spinal pain can be, especially if a full examination and X-rays have indicated the spine was essentially fine. I have listened to the frustrations of many patients who were treated by sincere doctors with only temporary or no results from these spinal manifestations. The HHS tricked them, just as it had tricked me. Admittedly, on frequent occasions it continues to trick me!

NUTRITIONAL SUGGESTIONS FOR BACKACHE IMBALANCES

1. Always make sure, as well as you know how, that the stomach is down! (Refer to Chapter, "What Can Be Done?"')
2. Use natural digestive aids, such as H.H.S. Formula, Pan-Gest or some type of betaine hydrochloride formula.
3. Use the diet outlined in Chapter 34.

DAILY

1. Manganese Aspartate -- 3 tablets, 3x a day
2. White willow bark -- 3 tablets, 3x a day for inflammation.
3. Magnesium/Calcium supplement (ratio 2 to 1) -- 1 tablet, 3x a day
4. Vitamin E -- 800 IU a day
5. Butcher's Broom -- 2 capsules, 3x a day
6. Beta Carotene -- 50,000 IU a day
7. Cherry Gold -- 6X a day (made for all structural problems and pain)
8. Minotaur--(a powder containing Creatine Monohydrate, Glutamine, Glucosamine Sulphate, and MSM) Take 1+ teaspoon daily. Mostly for men. Refer to catalog for more information.
9. Myo-Majestic--(a powder containing Creatine Monohydrate, Glutamine, Glucosamine Sulphate, MSM, Leucine, Isoleucine, and Valine) Take 1+ teaspoon daily. For men and women
10. Myo-My! -- (a powder containing Glutamine, Leucine, Isoleucine, and Valine) Take 1 teaspoon a day. For men and women
11. Glucosamine Sulphate -- 3x a day, 500 mg. each
12. Chondrotin Sulphate -- 3x a day

Chapter 21

ARTHRITIS AND ARTHRITIC TENDENCIES

Arthritis has an impressive link with the Hiatal Hernia Syndrome (HHS). If we allow the body, even unknowingly, to slowly starve because nutrients have failed to reach the cells by improper digestion and assimilation, the following happens: The body searches other areas of itself looking for these vital nutrients. The singular genetic prime directive is programmed into it: "Survival at all costs!"

Two primary elements the body must seek are calcium and protein:

1. **The body contains and must utilize more calcium than any other mineral.** Almost all of the calcium (two to three pounds) is found in the bones and teeth. The robbing process usually starts in the outer bones first. These are, of course, the hands and feet. Secondly, there is a noticeable overall demineralization (thinning) of the amount of calcium in all the bones, including the teeth. Even worse, after the body has taken the calcium needed from, let's say, the spine, it often doesn't utilize it properly. At this point the blood becomes more alkaline than it should be. Yet, the blood must remain in the right balance or it cannot hold its serum calcium within the bloodstream. Thus, calcium accumulates in places where it cannot be utilized. We often call these "arthritic spurs."

2. **Much of the body is actually protein:** a) Hormones; b) Genes; c) Secretions of the thyroid and pituitary; d) Insulin; e) Antibodies; f) Enzymes; g) Hemoglobin; h) Heart; i) Eyes; j) Liver; k) Kidneys. Skin and hair are 98% protein.

Look what happens when the HHS is present. It disrupts protein assimilation. To survive, the body robs this protein from within its own storage, thus weakening all the glands, organs and skin levels that desperately need protein to repair and sustain them.

Arthritic spurs are like having money in the bank and no check book to get it out. Since so much interference with digestion and assimilation renders bones thinner and thinner, and more and more brittle, our excess unobtainable bank account (arthritic spurs) grows larger. This causes nerve impairment and tissue inflammation. The ultimate result-- Pain!

Another phenomenon occurs. Many times the pains felt are not truly arthritis, but only arthritic tendencies. In my experience this is most often caused by adrenal insufficiency (sluggishness) and acid waste products which accumulate between the tissues. This produces aching in certain joints or, depending upon individual body chemistry, you just might "ache all over." I have seen this condition mistaken for *fibromyalgia* many times because of the similarity of the symptom patterns. (See my book, "Alkalize or Die".)

If there is achiness and pain, which has progressed to actual bone thinning, we always come back to the same point: The initial problem that links the causes together is the Hiatal Hernia Syndrome.

NUTRITIONAL SUGGESTIONS FOR ARTHRITIC TENDENCIES
(This is a very basic list.)
1. Always make sure, as well as you're able, that the stomach is down! (Refer to Chapter: "What Can Be Done?")
2. Use natural digestive aids, such as H.H.S. Formula, Pan-Gest or some type of betaine hydrochloride formula.
3. Use the diet outlined in Chapter 34.

DAILY
1. Bromelain (a pineapple enzyme) -- 8 tablets a day. This supplement has been shown to reduce swelling and inflammation in the soft tissues and joints affected by arthritis.
2. Vitamin C -- 3000 to 7000 mg. or Complete C -- 5 to 7 a day.
3. Potassium Aspartate or Orotate -- 500 mg. or Potassium Penetrator -- 1 to 2 a day.
4. Heated castor oil packs on affected areas, 45 min. a day.
5. Linseed oil -- 200 mg. a day.

6. Alfalfa tablets -- about 10 a day
7. B-6 --100 mg.
8. Pantothenic acid -- 100 mg. -- 3x a day
9. B-Complex -- high potency --3x a day or Bee Powerful 4 a day or B-Well -- 3 teas. daily
10. Vitamin E --up to 1000 IU
11. Tablets of sea vegetables -- 6 a day. (Wachter's brand is my favorite.)
12. Butcher's Broom -- 2 capsules, 3x a day
13. Magnesium/Calcium (ratio 2 to 1) -- 1 tablet, 3x a day or Magnesium Penetrator -- 2 in the morning and 2 at lunch and Calcium Penetrator -- 2+ at bedtime
14. Cherry Gold -- 9 to 12 a day. Made especially for arthritic imbalances
15. In-Sync-- 6 to 12 a day. Made especially for all types of pain syndromes, including arthritic imbalances.

Chapter 22

TEMPORO-MANDIBULAR JOINT IMBALANCES
(TMJ)

This intricate little joint plays a very important role in our lives. (See Diagram #11) Unless it operates properly, it isn't possible to eat well. There may be a clicking in your head each time you open your mouth. There may even be constant headaches. Imagine my surprise when I discovered several cases where patients with temporo-mandibular joint pain said, "My jaw stopped hurting and didn't bother me anymore until my stomach went up again."

Diagram #11

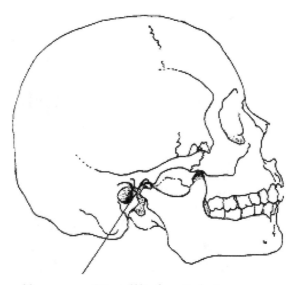

Temporo-Mandibular Joint

One possibility for this is the pathway taken by the stomach meridian in Chinese medicine. In part, it traces up the line of the mandible. The acupuncture points GB2 and

SI19 are right on top of the TMJ!

An interesting case, Mrs. C., came to me complaining of TMJ pain, various spinal ailments and stomach problems. I adjusted her spine, but the TMJ pain and stomach problem lingered. Not being a dentist I didn't initially look at the TMJ, for normally dentists file the teeth, supply a splint, or even surgically break the jaw to treat this problem. However, I corrected the HHS and was truly amazed when she told me of immediate relief in her TMJ as well. The pain returned only when she felt her stomach go up and her stomach problems recurred!

Another case: Mr. H. came to me with chronic tic-douloureux ("tic" for short), which is a highly painful problem that causes an intense jabbing pain in the face area. On examination, I found that the TMJ was misaligned. I worked with his neck, and he reported feeling much better and that the "tic" had stopped. Several weeks later he came in again, saying it had returned and that it had started when his stomach "felt funny and got upset." I examined him and found HHS. I corrected it and the "tic" stopped. Somehow (and I don't pretend to know how), these two conditions are equated.

Sometimes I think the HHS is too big for me. I sit back and wonder where it will stop. How long before the physiology of "the mother of all illness" is thoroughly and seriously explored? Discovery of TMJ involvement with the HHS leaves me in a quandary. All I can say to you, layperson and professional alike, is "**Correct the HHS and see if it alleviates pain-- any pain, anywhere in the body!**"

NUTRITIONAL SUGGESTIONS FOR TMJ IMBALANCES

1. Always make sure, as well as you're able, that the stomach is down! (Refer to the chapter: "What Can Be Done?")
2. Use natural digestive aids, such as H.H.S. Formula, Pan-Gest or some type of betaine hydrochloride formula.
3. Use the diet outlined in Chapter 34.

DAILY

1. Manganese Aspartate -- 3 tablets, 2x a day
2. B-Complex -- 3 tablets, 3x a day
3. White Willow bark -- (for inflammation) -- 2 tablets, 3x a day

4. Fennel Seed Caps. -- 1 cap. - 3X a day.
5. Cherry Gold -- 6X a day for joint and connective tissue pain.
6. In-Sync -- 6+ a day. For all types of pain syndromes.
7. Minotaur - (a powder containing Creatine Monohydrate, Glutamine, Glucosamine Sulphate, and MSM). Take 1+ teaspoon a day. Mostly for men. Refer to catalog for more information.
8. Myo-Majestic -- (a powder containing Creatine Monohydrate, Glutamine, Glucosamine Sulphate, MSM, Leucine, Isoleucine, and Valine) Take 1+ teaspoon a day For men and women.
9. Myo-My! -- (a powder containing Glutamine, Isoleucine, Leucine, and Valine. For men and women.
10. Glucosamine Sulphate -- 3X a day, 500 mg each.
11. Chondrotin Sulphate -- 3X a day.

Chapter 23

EAR IMBALANCES

"How can my stomach affect my *ears?*" Remember the vagus nerve? There is a branch of the vagus that goes to the ear! Remember when I said that the stomach goes up and pinches the vagus at the stomach level e.g., Hiatal Hernia Syndrome? When that nerve is pinched, it produces an acidic reaction. This creates distress throughout all of the surrounding cranial nerves. The eighth cranial nerve right there too. This nerve controls hearing. Whatever affects the vagus will indirectly affect the eighth cranial nerve.

Diagram #12

There are two important openings in your mouth that extend from the ears. They are called the Eustachian tubes. (See Diagram #12.) They serve as a drainage system for the ears. This drainage system stops up, what happens to the ears? Infection, pain, dizziness and sometimes a loss of hearing results because the pressure of the infected mucous pushes from the middle ear onto the inner ear. If this nerve pressure on the hearing nerve (8th cranial nerve) is not removed, then actual hearing loss may begin.

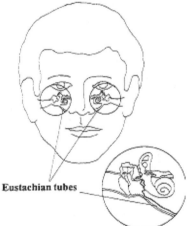

Eustachian tubes

When the HHS is corrected the Eustachian tubes sometimes open, which empties all the garbage out of the middle ear and releases the pressure on the inner ear as well. The inner ear is the one area that determines the body's ability to orient itself in space.

For instance, when Mrs. H came in she said that she constantly had to move some part of her body to orient herself in space. In her case there was a definite HHS. I corrected this and the lack of orientation completely disappeared. I was astounded. I have seen several such cases and for a long time found great difficulty understanding how it could happen.

I have since learned from a professional who works with children who have certain learning disabilities that these children always had to move "as if trying to orient themselves to where they were." Her report indicates to me that the presence of the HHS could account for this.

Obviously, this is another area that deserves research. Perhaps someone who is reading this book will do it. Again, I am not stating that the HHS causes ear problems. I am saying that when the vagus nerve is pinched, it produces acidity in the body, and this acidity possibly causes a constriction of the Eustachian Tubes as well as an indirect effect on the hearing nerve. Further, the garbage that doesn't drain out presses on the inner ear and this can create an ear problem, with resultant dizziness and disorientation.

NUTRITIONAL SUGGESTIONS FOR EAR IMBALANCES
1. Always make sure, as well as you're able, that the stomach is down! (Refer to the chapter: "What Can Be Done?")
2. Use natural digestive aids, such as H.H.S. Formula, Pan-Gest or some type of betaine hydrochloride formula.
3. Use the diet outlined in Chapter 34.

DAILY
1. Use 1 to 2 drops of either of these oils, or make a formula from equal parts of same: a) Castor oil; b) Tea Tree Oil; or c) use cinnamon oil alone.
2. Put Swedish Bitters on a piece of cotton, place in ears and leave it in overnight.
3. Use Disinfect. A preparation of the above oils plus eucalyptus and clove oils.

94

Chapter 24

HOARSENESS

Quite surprisingly one day as I listened to the after reports of HHS treatment for Mr. R., he mentioned, "Oh yes, and my hoarseness is better." Mr. R. had a chronic case of hoarseness that nothing medical or natural seemed to have given any relief.

Understandably curious, I searched the physiology texts once again for a possible clue.

The vagus nerve, our wandering friend, has a rather large branch right into the laryngeal plexus (throat area). As a result when other patients came in with this condition, I began to work vigorously on the HHS. Thereafter, their hoarseness improved. Some people improved only a little and some dramatically. I speculate the HHS is part of the cause for hoarseness for two reasons:

1. When the stomach ascends, it sometimes mechanically kinks the esophagus and manifests as irritation in the throat area.

2. The vagus nerve, being pinched by the HHS at the stomach, displays additional irritation into the laryngeal plexus of some individuals. This could lead to hoarseness.

I feel that "the mother of all illness", the HHS, could cause hoarseness. I am not referring to the kind of hoarseness you get by screaming your brains out at a football game. That is from overuse. I am talking about the chronic type that does not go away. I am stating that, clinically, I have watched hoarseness improve with HHS correction in certain cases. Since there are two possible reasons for hoarseness as a result of HHS involvement, is it so far fetched simply to work on your stomach as is given in this book and see if you improve as well?

NUTRITIONAL RECOMMENDATIONS FOR HOARSENESS

1. Always make sure, as well as you're able, that the stomach is down! (Refer to the chapter: "What Can Be Done?")

2. Use natural digestive aids, such as H.H.S. Formula, Pan-Gest or some type of betaine hydrochloride formula.

3. The Recipe is an all-natural liquid food supplement for coughing problems which is sometimes effective for hoarseness.

4. Racket-Free is an all natural liquid for snoring and asthmatic attacks that restrict the windpipe. It is also very soothing for hoarseness.

5. Another effective aid in these situations, use a mixture of these oils in equal parts: a) Peppermint oil; b) Eucalyptus oil; c) Juniper berry oil (can be omitted if difficult to get). Rub this mixture on the throat 3 times a day.

Chapter 25

PREMENSTRUAL SYNDROME IMBALANCES

For some women, Premenstrual Syndrome (PMS) can be a truly incapacitating state of affairs. It produces fatigue, irritability, sometimes utter depression, and an inability to cope with life for one or two weeks prior to actual menstruation. Their tension levels send them to doctor after doctor. When no medical help seems to work, they seek counseling or psychiatry. They will also try diet and nutritional supplements without satisfactory results. As a matter of fact, I have seen many cases of very determined women who have gone all three routes for help.

How this problem ties in with the Hiatal Hernia Syndrome (HHS) is most interesting. PMS is, in my opinion, another spin-off of hypoglycemia (low blood sugar). As hypoglycemia reaches a moderate level, PMS begins. The two are in the same immediate family. When care is taken to control the HHS and digestive enzymes are given, I find that a true change takes place. The prescribed diet, heretofore only partially successful, starts working so that vitamins and minerals begin to reach their proper cellular level for maintaining proper energy.

Remember the word "hypochondria" comes from the Greek word meaning "upper abdomen." Today, it connotes anxiety, tension, neurosis, fears and phobias. Also note that the area for the hiatal hernia is the "upper abdomen!" If the local health care professional doesn't spot PMS and calls you a hypochondriac, think of the possibility that the HHS is present.

Further, with PMS -- even after the Hiatal Hernia Syndrome is controlled and assimilation of nutrients is better-- I find it wise to prescribe specific vitamins and minerals. Since PMS is caused primarily by an imbalance of estrogen/progesterone in the body, we must be sure that after the low blood sugar condition is responding, the body is also receiving the correct amounts of Vitamin B-6, Vitamin E,

Calcium, Bee Pollen, and other hormonal components which are necessary for the rebalancing of this problem.

Again we find the "insidious link," the HHS, disrupting other biochemical functions and eventually causing them to go awry. This time it was women. Read on, my male friends; your time is coming, too.

NUTRITIONAL SUGGESTIONS FOR PREMENSTRUAL SYNDROME (PMS)

1. Always make sure, as well as you're able, that the stomach is down! (Refer to the chapter, "What Can Be Done?")
2. Use natural digestive aids, such as H.H.S. Formula, Pan-Gest or some type of betaine hydrochloride formula.
3. Use the diet outlined in Chapter 34.

DAILY

1) Vitamin B-6 -- 100 mg. 3x a day for one week before the menstrual cycle, then drop down to 50 mg. 3x a day.
2) Raw adrenal extract - 1 tablet, 3x a day or Feel Good -- 1-2X a day.
3) Raw ovarian extract -- 1 tablet, 3x a day or Women's Booster -- 1-3X a day.
4) Evening Primrose oil or Linseed oil -- 6x a day.
5) Potassium Penetrator -- 2 a day.
6) Vitamin E -- up to 2000 IU a day.
7) Dong Quai -- 500 mg. 3x a day.
8) Raw Thymus extract -- 3 tablets, 3x a day. (Recent information suggests that PMS is partly due to bacterial infections. Thymus extract will balance this infection and greatly strengthen the weakened immune system.)
9) I strongly recommend the following at the onset of menses:
   a) Drink strong Valerian root tea each night from three days before onset until cycle ends.
   b) Take an Epsom salt bath nightly and maybe another during the day.
   c) Use a hot castor oil pack on your abdomen each night to ease cramping. This procedure will many times help the cramping to be of much less duration and severity.
10) Fennel Seed Caps -- 1 cap. 3X a day.

11) Protone-- a very potent progesterone cream. Rub a dab on end of finger onto ovary area 2X a day.

Chapter 26

CANDIDA ALBICANS IMBALANCES

One of the health problems that have come to the attention of health practitioners nationwide in recent years is a condition called Candida Albicans. It is a fungus that is always in the body. When there are biochemical imbalances it multiplies, causing an unbelievably long list of ill-health involvements. It is a great mimicker. Traditional medicine recognizes it as a cause for vaginal problems. The tremendous body of research on this problem shows that not only vaginal problems are a part of this infection.

Other symptoms and conditions it produces are:
1) Fatigue or lethargy, "drained feeling"
2) Poor memory, "spacey feeling"
3) Depression
4) Numbness, burning or tingling
5) Muscle aches, weakness, or paralysis
6) Pain and/or swelling in joints
7) Abdominal pain
8) Constipation
9) Diarrhea
10) Bloating
11) Troublesome vaginal discharge
12) Persistent vaginal burning or itching
13) Prostatitis
14) Impotence
15) Loss of sexual desire
16) Endometriosis
17) Cramps and/or other menstrual irregularities
18) Premenstrual tension
19) Spots in front of eyes
20) Erratic vision

The above is a list of major symptoms. There are many minor symptoms as well.

Obviously large numbers of people, both men and women, have this problem. Currently, there are several good books on this subject. One of the most authoritative is by William Crook, M.D., entitled *The Yeast Connection*. If you have any of these symptoms, you might do well to consult someone in the health care field who is knowledgeable about Candida.

Let us examine this widespread problem in relationship to the Hiatal Hernia Syndrome (HHS). Healthcare practitioners from several fields all agree that in such cases the immune system of the body has become sluggish. This causes the natural checks and balances of the body to under-function; consequently, there is a proliferation of this stubborn fungus, Candida Albicans.

Now go back a little further. What causes the auto-immune system to become sluggish and under-function? Again, it is that proper digestion and assimilation have caused a situation of poor nutrition to occur in the body. This leads to low blood sugar, poor adrenal function, and many other conditions we have discussed.

What causes the body to digest and assimilate improperly? Again, could it not be that the stomach has gone up just slightly, interfering with vagus nerve function and hydrochloric acid production? If you refer to Diagram #3, you will remember just how extensive the vagus nerve is. Would this not cause poor assimilation of food, which leads to immune system under-function, and finally the imbalances in body chemistry that end up with increased overproduction of Candida Albicans?

Clinical experience suggests to me that the HHS exists prior to the overproduction of Candida Albicans. In my practice, I have found the treatment to be the same. That is, the HHS and Candida Albicans must be treated simultaneously. There is justification for this. If you have a fungus infection and only treat the HHS, the infection will not improve for long and neither will the HHS. All the reasons for this are not clear. One hypothesis: it is the fungus that causes irritating excess mucous in the whole system, as part of the body's attempt to control the Candida. This excess mucous accumulates in the esophageal hiatus - the very place the HHS is manifesting!

This aggravates the esophagus and stomach, causing an *upward contraction. The "insidious link" is at it again!*

101

From here problems just build, as has been previously discussed. There is hope. Success with Candida Albicans is a proven fact. It does take time. Discuss this with your nutritionally minded health professional. But please don't let him forget that the HHS may be lurking also.

NUTRITIONAL SUGGESTIONS FOR CANDIDA ALBICANS IMBALANCES

1) Always make sure, as well as you're able, that the stomach is down! (Refer to the chapter, "What Can Be Done?")
2) Use natural digestive aids, such as H.H.S. Formula, Pan-Gest or some type of betaine hydrochloride formula.
3) Use the diet outlined in Chapter 34.

DAILY

Many books have this information available. However, I will add a few lesser known excellent candida killers. These are:

1) Pau d'Arco Tea -- drink 3 cups a day.
2) Myrrh tincture -- 10 drops, 3x a day.
3) Biotin -- 2000 mcgs. per day.
4) Caprylic Acid -- 3X a day with food.
5) Nutribiotic drops -- 3 a day in water.
6) A good acidophilus product -- 3 a day or Colonize -- 3 a day.
7) Fungal Foe -- Made specifically for all fungal imbalances and Candida Albicans in particular. Take 6 a day and more if your health practitioner is monitoring you.
8) Free Breath -- although made for lung problems, it really goes after Candida very aggressively. -- 6 a day.
9) Zymex (from Standard Process Labs) -- 9 a day.
10) Black Walnut Hulls -- 4 a day.
11) Reduce fruit, starch and sugar drastically. Candida loves fruit.

Chapter 27

PROSTATE IMBALANCES

I was floored to discover a definite relationship between the Hiatal Hernia Syndrome (HHS) and prostate problems. The "insidious link" completes its circuitry at this point. The tie in is through our old friend, the vagus nerve. As is pictured in Diagram # 3, the vagus nerve intersects with the pelvic nerve, which eventually leads to the prostate gland. An interesting clue was a mild case of diarrhea a patient experienced after the prostate started acting up. I then discovered this in other cases. Upon further investigation, I found the HHS present with many prostate sufferers.

I listened as several prostate gland victims told me about their desire to push downward from the HHS point into the prostate area. Although they didn't know the significance of that point, pressing downward gave them some temporary relief. Upon correcting the HHS, I have observed that several men reported "better feeling, more together, less aching, less swelling" in the prostate area.

Could it be that the HHS is causing some type of nerve energy blockage to the prostate through the vagus nerve's being pinched by the HHS? Could it be the HHS definitely affects proper food absorption and precious minerals like zinc are not reaching the prostate?

From my viewpoint, both of these play a part in chronic cases of prostatitis. Drugs help the prostate symptoms, but the causes are not addressed, else why would chronic prostatitis keep coming back even after therapy?

I contend that the HHS is an "insidious link" that plays a part in its perpetuation.

NUTRITIONAL SUGGESTIONS FOR PROSTATE IMBALANCES

1) Always make sure, as well as you're able, that the stomach is down! (Refer to Chapter, "What Can Be Done?")
2) Use natural digestive aids, such as H.H.S. Formula,

        Pan-Gest or some type of betaine hydrochloride formula.

3)   Use the diet outlined in Chapter 34.

DAILY

1)   Zinc Orotate -- 60 mg. a day or Zinc Penetrator -- 1 to 2 a day

2)   Vitamin E -- 800 IU a day

3)   Protector (made for prostate imbalances) -- 1 tablet, 3x a day. This food supplement has the herb Saw Palmetto in it as one of the primary ingredients. Take more depending upon how advanced the imbalance is occurring. Check with your health practitioner and get dosages.

4)   Butcher's Broom -- 2 capsules, 3x a day

5)   Herbal laxatives and colonics are suggested to reduce pressure from the colon.

6)   Can-Clear -- has definite prostate support and was made for this, but it is also a laxative. Use common sense about the amount -- 2 at bed. If you have diarrhea, do not use this product.

Chapter 28

EPILEPSY IMBALANCES

This is one of the most fascinating considerations yet presented! The Hiatal Hernia Syndrome (HHS) may play a part, even in epilepsy. Surprisingly, a very small percentage of this problem seems to lie in brain malfunction, although it is conventionally stated as being the primary cause.

The vagus nerve is pinched at the stomach level when the HHS is present. This causes the vagus to malfunction throughout the entire body. The branch of the vagus to the small intestines is no exception. It malfunctions, producing an acid state, which hinders proper absorption of food and somewhat restricts the circulation of blood in the area of the small intestines. The small intestines are the restaurant for the body. They take digested food from the 'kitchen' and send it out for the whole body to be fed. When a lack of circulation occurs in the small intestines, a new situation presents itself.

There the tissue starts to adhere, or stick together, in areas where it is not supposed to. Over even a short period of time, this causes actual abnormal, tissue like formation called an adhesion (See Diagram #13.) Adhesions of this type can also

Diagram #13

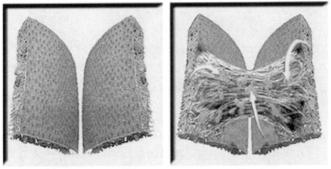

Normal Peritoneum	**Adhesion**
(Membrane	*(In The Abdomen Or Pelvic Area)*
Of The Abdominal Cavity)	

occur because of abdominal surgery or because of an injury to the area. In either case, the adhesion blocks the normal functioning of the small intestines. In addition to the adhesion, the nervous system is involved and pinched, causing a spasm in the smooth muscle of the intestines. This would not be so bad if the spasm just stayed in that area, but it doesn't. Through the nervous system, it causes the whole body to spasm. The seriousness of the adhesions in the small intestines generally determines how bad the spasms can be -- either small (petite mal) or large (grand mal).

Correction of just the HHS isn't enough in cases of epilepsy, but it can help. There are manipulations for the soft tissue that can help to free adhesions in the abdominal area. A chiropractor, osteopath, or massage therapist may know these techniques of manipulation. Certified Holographic Health Practitioners have checks for adhesions and may be able to at least offer some relief. Be sure to rub Campho-Heal or some other therapeutic oil known to help with adhesions on the abdominal cavity.

These new perspectives and techniques may assist in the reduction and control of the inscrutable threat posed by epilepsy.

NUTRITIONAL SUGGESTIONS FOR EPILEPSY
1) Always make sure, as well as you know how, that the stomach is down! (Refer to Chapter, "What Can Be Done?")
2) Use natural digestive aids, such as H.H.S. Formula, Pan-Gest or some type of betaine hydrochloride formula.
3) Use the diet outlined in Chapter 34.

DAILY
1) Thyroid extract, or Energy Up -- (1) 3X a day.
2) Vitamin E -- start with 100 IU. Over a three month period, increase to 2000 IU.
3) B-6 -- 100 mgs. 2x a day.
4) B-Complex -- 3x a day or B-Well -- 3 teas. a day.
5) Vitamin C -- 2000 mg. or Complete C -- 4 a day.
6) Zinc Orotate -- 30 mg. or Zinc Penetrator -- 1 a day.
7) Niacinamide -- 50 mg.
8) Magnesium/Calcium (ratio 2 to 1) -- 1 tablet, 3x a day or Magnesium Penetrator -- 2 in the morning and Calcium Penetrator -- 1 at bedtime.

9) Raw adrenal extract -- 3x a day, or Feel Good -- 3 a day.
10) Vitamin A -- beta carotene 25,000 IU.
11) EPA oils -- 1200 mg or Alpha-Omega -- 2 to 3 a day.
12) Check for intestinal parasites and worms. Epilepsy has been linked to these. Try Para-Go-Way if these are suspected or found. -- 9 a day
13) Swedish Bitters Compress applied to the base of the skull, nightly.
14) L-Tyrosine -- 2 (2X a day)
15) At Eez -- 2 at bed or at the first symptoms of seizure activity. Helps to repair and strengthen the nervous system.
16) Symmetry -- This food supplement is designed to support all kinds of nervous system imbalances. I have had success with it for this imbalance. - 3 to 6 a day. Check with your health practitioner for dosages.
17) L-Glutamine powder -- 2 teas. per day.

Chapter 29

CANCER IMBALANCES

The subject of cancer is one that brings with it a sense of foreboding and hopelessness. Although the incidence of gastrointestinal cancer is very high in comparison to other types of cancer, I make no claims here that the Hiatal Hernia Syndrome (HHS) is the cause. The premise is offered to show possible links between digestion and the chaos in the body called cancer.

If the body is being undernourished because it is not digesting and assimilating its food correctly, a pattern of chronic fatigue and low blood sugar symptoms will finally manifest. The by-products of improperly digested food in the system not only block up the small and large intestine and cause constipation, but also produce a far more imposing problem -- fermentation of the food. Cancer of any type proliferates in an environment of fermentation and anaerobic cell activity. The normal cell uses oxygen to assist in its replication. Anaerobic means that the cell multiplies without oxygen, by fermentation. This combination of anaerobic activity and fermentation provides an excessive amount of acidity for the cancer cells, which seem to flourish in this environment.

There is evidence to show that the body quite often produces cancerous cells to a small extent but readily destroys them because of its wonderful ability to monitor, maintain, and heal itself. A small scale example of this is warts. They are benign cancers that come and go many times without our conscious effort to remove them.

It stands to reason that as long as the immune system of the body is working properly and the energy of digestion is correct, we will have a basically cancer free body.

Now let me introduce the unsuspected factor, the HHS. Suppose Mr. H., a healthy, vital 30-year-old man with good digestion and assimilation suddenly has an accident in which he is hit in the stomach. This injury widens the esophageal hiatus, and the stomach ascends. Perhaps the only symptoms

Mr. H displays are tightness in the upper abdomen, a shortness of breath, and that nothing he eats seems to satisfy him.

Several months pass, and he starts to feel more and more fatigued. The shortness of breath persists. This is one of the classical symptoms of hiatal hernia. It occurs because the lungs are being crowded by the stomach ascension. The ability to fully oxygenate the blood by breathing deeply and freely into the abdomen is restricted. Remember that normal cell replication requires oxygen. Without oxygen, the cell reproduces itself by anaerobic (lack of oxygen) activity, which leads to cell mutation, or cancer.

Now let me add more factors to this picture. Poor digestion causes poor elimination. Mr. H. is retaining poisonous substances in his bowels too long. Some of these toxins seep back into the bloodstream. He feels even worse, partly because more of his food ferments than is digested. The other factor for a cancer environment is fermentation in which the cancer cell feeds and quickly multiplies. Mr. H. is starting to get worried. He feels run down and something in him just doesn't seem right. Let us assume this environment continues in his body for 10 years. Add to this daily stress and the lack of energy to handle normal stress, which creates more stress, fatigue and frustration. Also, throw in a moderate amount of refined processed "fast food", which is highly acid-forming. In these circumstances, Mr. H. is a prime target for cancer development.

DO ANY OF THESE CONDITIONS SOUND FAMILIAR?

I recently talked to a hospice worker. She reported her helplessness and distress, as she watched the last twenty cancer patients die. She stated empathically that they did not die of cancer, but starved to death!

What determines starvation? If you are eating well, how can you starve? It is simple. That is what this book is all about. If the stomach goes up (HHS), it does not digest and assimilate food well enough; consequently, you do indeed starve.

After years of observation, I am convinced that the body does not recognize malignant tumors as a threat. If this is the case, the immune system does not know how to deal with them and they grow without much opposition. In my opinion, the best way to deal with any form of cancer is to find a way to crack the shell of the pathogens and then the immune system could rebalance the exposed DNA.

It is common knowledge that we are still badly losing in the fight against cancer. This isn't the medical profession's fault. Daily acts of heroism in medicine are saving many potential cancer victims from an untimely death. Cancer is a challenge to everybody. No one has all the answers. Massive efforts are being made to conquer this enigma. I myself do not diagnose or treat any cancer, but I would not be surprised if the HHS were found in a very large number of those afflicted. At least, make sure "the mother of all illness" is under control if you find it.

(No nutritional suggestions are being made here, because many health books are available on this subject and professional guidance is recommended as well.)

Chapter 30

PREGNANCY

Pregnancy can be such a wonderful experience! There is excitement and joy, along with anticipation.

Unfortunately, many women report the distress during pregnancy that their stomach gives them. Sometimes the enlarged uterus crowds the stomach area and forces it upward. This, of course, can produce the Hiatal Hernia Syndrome (HHS).

I definitely find the HHS linked to morning sickness in the early stages of pregnancy. In the latter stages, when more distention of the abdomen exists, the stomach can still be moved into a better position. Try the milder techniques like stretching back before and after meals. Also, let someone else try putting hands on the HHS area for several minutes. The heat from the hands may relax the diaphragm, and the stomach will often drop enough to bring great relief.

Frequently, I hear women tell me that they carried little Johnny so high that from that time to this their "stomach just hasn't been right." Doctors, be sure to make this correction for new mothers! Husbands, do the same! Don't let the HHS plague your lovely wife or impair her ability to feel well throughout motherhood!

Chapter 31

CHILDREN

It is not uncommon for me to see children who have the Hiatal Hernia Syndrome (HHS). Just stop and think for a moment how often children are rolling and tumbling around. Hardly a day goes by that they don't get hit somewhere. In fact, it just may be that most of the problems adults have with their stomachs started when they were young. A good hit in the belly could easily trigger this problem.

A two-month-old boy was brought to me because he was having **colic** almost all the time. I did not think to look for the HHS as first and must admit that I was quite surprised when I did find it. After the correction was made, which at this age is easy and gentle, the colic stopped within one day and didn't return for about two weeks. Upon examining him I found the HHS again. I corrected it, and again the colic stopped.

This discovery in itself was very enlightening to me. I had always been taught: "It is normal for children to have colic." Now I feel this is not so, when looked at from this viewpoint. Many of an infant's problems occur in and through the stomach. Consider the HHS when your child is having a "stomach problem" or is even displaying hyperactivity.

Hyperactivity is a common complaint I hear from mothers. When childrens' digestive ability is compromised, they can develop symptoms of adrenal over-stimulation. This means a hyperactive state. You may be surprised, as I have been, when they calm so quickly after the correction of the HHS.

Is the HHS the only cause of stomach problems in children? No. In my experience, there is an undeniable "link." When digestion is disturbed, no matter at what age, trouble is brewing.

Chapter 32

CONDITIONS WHICH
MISLEAD IN DIAGNOSIS

There are four conditions that can markedly mislead in attempting to diagnose HHS problems as a principal causative factor. Do not take any of the first three lightly. Suggestions are given that may help you with the fourth one, as well.

1.   CONGESTIVE HEART FAILURE

This is a condition that can mimic the HHS and should be carefully watched. It is well to suspect this condition in any older person who shows HHS symptoms and chest congestion. Often in its initial stages, congestive heart failure may be completely overlooked or be mis-diagnosed as pneumonia. If you should have any reason whatsoever to suspect this condition, alert a medical doctor immediately. In these cases the HHS can occur and even when you correct it, the stomach will only stay down for a very short period because of the fluid in the lower lung areas.

2.   ENLARGED ORGANS

A very difficult condition to deal with is enlarged organs, such as the liver or spleen. These will press against the stomach and force it through the already weakened diaphragm. Usually these organs can be felt by applying gentle hand pressure to the painful area. Again, it is very important to get medical attention as soon as you suspect this condition. Even if the HHS is present, you will not be able to keep it under control in this situation.

Whether digestive disorders caused by the HHS led to these conditions is a moot question when the situation becomes this serious. Just get medical attention.

3.   FOOD POISONING

The topic of food poisoning is a tricky one. I am greatly alarmed how often food sensitivity or poisoning happens now in comparison to a few years ago. Many of the symptoms I usually see are intense stomach area pain and/or vomiting. The stomach will always be forced up in these situations because of the highly acidic effect of poison on the system and the spasming of stomach muscles, and thus give all appearances of being a confirmed HHS.

Although you may be able to get the stomach into place with the techniques given in the next chapter, again I advise you not to try in such acute cases unless you have quite a bit of experience with this particular problem. I find that the stomach will not stay down more than a few minutes until the food substance in question leaves the upper stomach or is vomited up.

You may try using charcoal capsules, which work extremely well, to help at such times. If you think you have been poisoned by something you have eaten, consider medical assistance.

4.   THE HHS VIRUS

At first I thought this was the identified Epstein-Barr virus, but I have since ruled this out. This is a treacherous masquerader. I have agonized over how to reach and aid the person with this unrecognized virus. This can be undoubtedly our single greatest foe in the battle against the "insidious link" of HHS.

It can have an onset, then lie dormant for periods of time, and emerge again in a lesser or greater way. This can go on from 12 to 15 years if not eradicated. The way it emerges generally causes an overall fatigue, but perhaps with no sniffles or other viral signs. It does, however, affect the stomach by causing definite stomach ascension. Even consistent manipulation or exercises don't help for more than a few moments. In the cases of this nature, no drug seems to help. Since very little true digestion can occur because the stomach is up, I find the victim going very quickly into low blood sugar.

What can be done? The frustration of watching nothing work is unbearable. By itself the virus doesn't seem to be particularly fatal, and it will finally subside; then the stomach will stabilize, and the victim and doctor will feel it is over. Unfortunately, this virus only submerges, waiting for another chance. Generally, I find that the virus runs in cycles.

In the case of Ms. H. it subsided, then re-emerged with a vengeful fury exactly three years later. It may mimic mononucleosis, but blood work will show negative. The involvement of the stomach will be subtle with some people, but is usually a major complaint and can lead to acid reflux and vomiting of food.

Although the method of treatment I adopt may appear different, I ask that it be considered. It dates back 100 years to the time in India when color therapy was understood, as was the use of gems in relation to healing. To my knowledge, there is no other way to reach this foe. I investigated the available traditional and nontraditional therapies before this one was employed. It is as follows:

Place 2 parts pure spring water and 1 part pure grain alcohol in a clear glass jar with an amethyst (purple) crystal. Let the jar stay in full sun for a minimum of five hours. Take at least 1 tablespoon twice a day. This seems to work miracles. The idea is to get the ultra-violet light into the water. This is not such a far-fetched idea when you realize violet light is used by dermatologists to help treat skin infections in some cases. Ultra-violet light can definitely affect this virus.

I have encountered all four of the above conditions. They are frustrating and can be very dangerous. Get medical attention if there are questions about what you are dealing with and if the symptoms sounds like those described.

Chapter 33

HIATAL HERNIA SYNDROME AND DRUGS

The classes of drugs that deal with the symptoms of a Hiatal Hernia Sydrome are among the largest and most popular in the world. This fits very well into my clinical prediction that about 85% of the population experiences the effects of the Hiatal Hernia Syndrome at one time or another.

Tagamet®: even in the *Physician's Desk Reference,* is highly lauded. This is one of the drug industry's stars.

This is written chemically as: N'-cyano-N-methyl-N'[2-] [5-methyl-1H-imidozol-4-yl) methyl]thio]-ethyl] - guanidine - for which there is no biochemical formulation in our body. Does this sound inviting?

Just exactly what does Tagamet® do? It decreases the amount of gastric (acid) secretions in the stomach. It is widely used in the treatment of ulcers. In some cases there is little doubt that Tagamet® does help; however, I see many patients whom it does not help.

In the previous chapter on ulcers I explained my findings that the Hiatal Hernia Syndrome (HHS) was always present when ulceration occurred. If the HHS exists, whether Tagamet® slows down acid production or not, the problem is still there. The ulcer is only the result. Curing a symptom doesn't solve the problem.

There appears to be even more than just acid production that is slowed down as a result of Tagamet® use. A most wonderful substance in our body called "lymph" helps to carry off the many used and poisonous products from our cells and blood. Without proper functioning of the lymphatic system we would soon die. Tagamet® slows this flow of lymph down by drying up portions of it and interfering with its production in the liver.

I have seen Tagamet® given in many cases for increased burning (also an HHS symptom) where there was no ulceration. Note that other ways of dealing with this problem are discussed in the chapter, "What You Can Do For Yourself". The following is a list of side effects of Tagamet®: *Minor side-effects*: Diarrhea, dizziness, headache, muscle pain.

Major side effects: Easy bruising, confusion, fever, hair loss, increased breast size, impotence, jaundice, palpitations, rash, sore throat, weakness.

I'm not saying that Tagamet® or drug therapy has no place. I'm only asking: "Why not try more conservative, more natural therapies first? If they don't work, and the correction of the HHS doesn't help, then consider drug therapy."

There is another point for attention here. Many times the excess acid in the stomach is merely a reaction to an increase of bile that is back washed into the upper part of the stomach as explained in the chapter on ulcers. (See Diagram #6) This means that to begin with there was not enough hydrochloric acid in the stomach for proper food breakdown. If this already failing function is even further suppressed, are we truly getting to the problem or only covering it up for a more serious problem later?

Taking this argument a step further, even if the problem were not the HHS, do we truly want to suppress hydrochloric acid production considering its important place in digestion and assimilation? What happens to food when it doesn't break down properly because an ulcer drug is interfering with the initial phase of digestion? Wouldn't it be wiser to work with natural substances to heal the ulcer and balance the flow of hydrochloric acid?

What about those people who don't even have an ulcer at this time, only acid reflux? What is drug suppression of hydrochloric acid doing here? If the body doesn't get the nutrition it needs from the food which is eaten, then be very aware that the body will try to fill its needs by feeding on itself. This, as has been stated before, causes a multitude of different illnesses.

Valium®: 7-chloro- 1, 2-dihydro -1-methyl- 5 phenyl- 2'H-1, 4-benzodiaze-pin-2-one.

Although this is not a drug that is prescribed specifically for hiatal hernia and acid reflux, I feel that its wide use as a relaxant should be examined here in light of our previous findings.

When the HHS occurs, there is a tremendous amount of

117

anxiety produced. (See the chapter: "Mental Distress Imbalances".) Remember that even the point of distress above the stomach is in the area called "hypochondria," which is where the term "hypochondriac" comes from. (See Diagram #15 of HHS point)

It should be said that I have found that when the muscles have been relaxed through the use of Valium®, in some cases the HHS corrects itself. In other words the stomach drops down into proper place. Valium® has an addictive nature according to the *Physician's Desk Reference*. Taking Valium into an already upset system for long periods of time to help the stomach stay down has side effects.

Mrs. P. came in with high blood pressure, mental confusion and a great deal of shakiness. Her past pattern had been days in intensive care taking Valium® injections. I found the lurking HHS and corrected it. All symptoms stopped and she left the office without high blood pressure, mental confusion or shakiness.

In light of current national and world stresses there is small wonder that so many individuals suffer stomach problems and turn to the crutch of palliative drugs. Since this is the case, is it so far-fetched that HHS therapy offers a practical solution? Is the Hiatal Hernia Syndrome such an alien concept? Clinical experience with this pandemic problem certainly indicates that the HHS should be dealt with first, then other methods pursued only after it is definitely ruled out.

Reglan®: This is chemically: 4 -amino -5-chl oro -N- [2 - die tthylamin o) ethyl] – 2-methoxybenzamide monohydrochloride monohydrate - (Reglan®).

This drug is used to increase gastric contractions, relax the pyloric sphincter, and accelerate the movement of food on through to the small intestine. Also, it allows the lower esophageal sphincter to relax.

The real problem with Reglan® is that along with its ability to speed food down and along the intestinal tract, it nullifies digestive enzymes. This means that food is not digesting properly again, and one can expect more complications further down the line. It is true that this drug helps to relieve nausea or vomiting by allowing the food to get into the small intestine quicker. The feeling of fullness, nausea and vomiting are also symptoms of the HHS! You might want to check for its presence and correct it first.

Donnazyme®: This is an honest attempt to alleviate stomach problems. It is aimed at helping to increase digestive enzymes by supplying some of them. It also contains belladonna alkaloids like phenobarbital. Phenobarbital, according to the *Physician's Desk Reference,* may be habit forming. It further states these adverse reactions: xerostomia, urinary hesitancy, blurred vision, tachycardia, palpitation, mydriasis, cycloplegia, increased ocular tension, loss of taste sense, headache, nervousness, drowsiness, weakness, dizziness, insomnia, nausea, vomiting, impotence, suppression of lactation, constipation, bloated feeling, musculoskeletal pain and severe allergic reaction or drug idiosyncrasies, including "anaphylaxis, urticaria and other dermal manifestations, and decreased sweating."

If the HHS is occurring and the stomach is up, hydrochloric acid is too low, so we are still missing the main part of the problem as far as digestion is concerned. We want to have enough hydrochloric acid to break down the food in the first phase of our digestion.

Zantac® is another drug that inhibits gastric secretions. It creates the same interference as the others do. Indeed, the list of side effects in Zantac® is rather impressive. A few are headaches, dizziness, insomnia, vertigo, constipation, diarrhea, nausea, vomiting, abdominal discomfort and rash.

Pepcid®: works by the inhibition of hydrochloric acid. I have rarely seen it help dramatically and side effects exist: fever, headache, dizziness, constipation, diarrhea, fatigue, palpitations, nausea, vomiting, dry mouth, bronchospasm, alopecia, acne, rash, dry skin, and tinnitus.

Prilosec®: This was the drug of choice for years and now has been deemed safe enough to sell over the counter. It is one of the primary drugs of choice for gastroesophageal reflux. It has so many side effects that use is not recommended for long. Besides reducing our much-needed hydrochloric acid, it has been recently documented to decrease B-12 absorption in healthy subjects by over 300%.

Nexium®: This is the next generation of the Prilosec® line. It is called the "purple pill". Reactions in the body are similar to Prilosec® and the results are about the same except they appear to act faster. This still does not address the HHS. It just covers up the problem. After realigning the HHS into its proper position, these medicines could even work better, if they were needed at all.

A drug is not food, and in my opinion, the body will not be tricked too long. The nutritional food supplementation mentioned throughout this book is not harmful in any way to the body. There are certainly times, however, when drug therapy is necessary. In light of this review it is now prudent to ask: Would correction of the HHS be preferable to taking drugs?

Chapter 34

Diet

The most important key to avoiding the HHS is adopting a proper diet. It is a brave and sometimes difficult thing to change your way of eating. If you have the Hiatal Hernia Syndrome, you should give it your best effort.

The intent here is to give you what is basic and effective, yet simple and usable. You can adopt these suggestions slowly without causing a stressful adjustment. Your body will help you with this. As certain poor dietary habits drop away, these new ones will replace them naturally and comfortably.

Above all, it is important to get as close as possible to 80% of your food from the alkaline-forming food list and only 20% from the acid-forming food list. Over a long period of time this 80% to 20% ratio has definitely proved to be the best for the body. More information about alkaline/acid forming biochemistry is available in my book Alkalize Or Die I have researched and compiled these lists to give you what I consider the most comprehensive ones available. Also included is a standard food combining chart. (See Diagram #14.)

SUGGESTIONS FOR HEALTHY EATING

1. Keep your meals simple -- 3 or 4 foods are enough. Eat more raw foods in the summer.
2. Don't mix fruits and vegetables at the same meal. Fresh fruits are digested rapidly (75-90 minutes), while meats, wheat, Brussels sprouts, and turnips can take up to 4 hours.
3. Avoid more than two high protein foods like beef and chicken at the same meal.
4. Avoid more than two starches, like potatoes and beets, at the same meal.
5. Omit refined foods and sweeteners! (White bread, white rice, white sugar, etc).
6. Try phasing out dairy products.
7. Avoid alcohol.

8. Don't cook with hardened vegetable oils.
9. Take digestive aids 5 minutes before each major meal.
10. Don't wash your food down with liquids. Let your food mix with saliva.
11. Drink 6-8 glasses of water a day, between meals.
12. Don't eat when you are anxious, angry, overheated, chilled, in high fever, or just not hungry.

Note: The absorption of vitamin B-12 is dependent on hydrochloric acid production. Certain drugs like Zantac®, Tagamet® and Pepsid®, block HCL production. Now that these drugs and their clones are over-the-counter, B-12 deficiencies will become even more widespread. A Vitamin B-12 deficiency can cause symptoms of fatigue, breathlessness, muscle weakness, and neurological symptoms.

The following ALKALINE/ACID-FORMING FOOD LIST found on the next page shows a representative list of foods that are either alkaline-forming or acid-forming in the system.

ALKALINE/ACID-FORMING FOOD LIST

The body seems to work best on a high ratio of alkaline-forming foods - those foods which give alkaline elements when broken down by digestion. A diet which contains 70-80% alkaline forming foods is ideal for healthful living.

FRUITS

Acid - Blueberries, coconut, cranberries (unless mixed with ½ water), Damson plums, dried fruit, canned fruit, jams, jellies, sugared and sulphured fruits.
Alkaline - All other fresh fruits and fresh juices: Apples, apricots, avocado, bananas, berries, cherries, currants, figs, grapes, grapefruit, kiwi, lemons, limes, melons, nectarine, oranges, papaya, peaches, pears, persimmons, pineapple, plum, pomegranate, prunes, pumpkin, raisins, raspberry, sour grape, strawberries, tangerines, tomatoes, watermelon.

VEGETABLES

Acid - Ginger, sweet potatoes.
Alkaline - All other fresh vegetables: artichokes, asparagus, bamboo shoots, beets, broccoli, brussels sprouts, cabbage, carrots, cauliflower, celery, collards, corn(sweet), cucumbers, daikon, dandelion greens, eggplant, endive, escarole, garlic,

horseradish, kale, kelp, leeks, lettuces, mushrooms, okra, olives, onions, parsley, parsnips, peas, peppers, potatoes (if eaten with skins), radishes, rhubarb, rutabaga, sauerkraut, spinach, summer squash, Swiss chard, taro, turnips, watercress, winter squash.

GRAINS

Acid - Barley, brown rice, oats, rye berries, and wheat berries.
Alkaline - Buckwheat, corn (dry), millet, quinoa. Any grain that is sprouted is alkaline.

MEATS/PROTEINS

Acid - Beef, fowl, game, lamb, pork, and other meats, fish, eggs, cheeses.
Alkaline - Acidophilus, raw milk, whey, yogurt (with no sugar).
Neutral - Butter, cream, margarine.

BEANS

Acid - Aduki, black, garbanzo, kidney, lentils, navy, red, soy, white and any other dried beans.
Alkaline - Green, lima, fresh peas, snap, soybeans, string, and all sprouted dry beans.

STARCHES

Acid - Bran, breads, cereals, cornstarch, crackers, custards, flours, oatmeal, pastries, popcorn, white rice, spaghetti.
Alkaline - Potatoes cooked and eaten with the peel.

NUTS

Acid - Cashews, filberts, macadamia, peanuts, pecans, pistachios, walnuts, water chestnuts and any nut that is toasted or cooked.
Alkaline - Almonds, Brazil, chestnuts, pignolias (pine nuts).

SEEDS

Acid - Alfalfa, chia, pumpkin, radish, sesame, sunflower.
Alkaline - All sprouted seeds.

Diagram #14

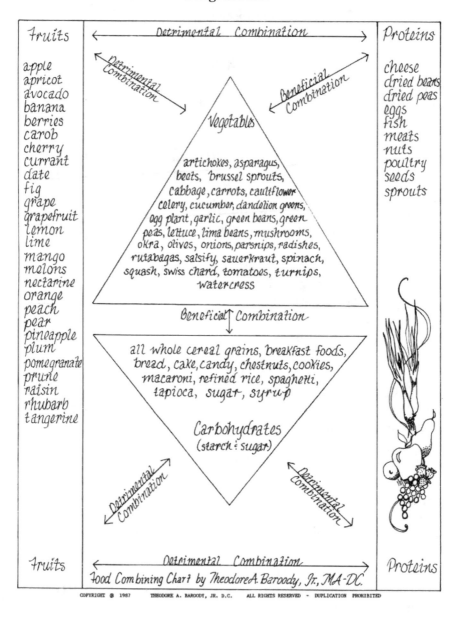

Fruits

apple
apricot
avocado
banana
berries
carob
cherry
currant
date
fig
grape
grapefruit
lemon
lime
mango
melons
nectarine
orange
peach
pear
pineapple
plum
pomegranate
prune
raisin
rhubarb
tangerine

Proteins

cheese
dried beans
dried peas
eggs
fish
meats
nuts
poultry
seeds
sprouts

← Detrimental Combination →

Detrimental Combination

Beneficial Combination

Vegetables

artichokes, asparagus,
beets, brussel sprouts,
cabbage, carrots, cauliflower,
celery, cucumber, dandelion greens,
egg plant, garlic, green beans, green
peas, lettuce, lima beans, mushrooms,
okra, olives, onions, parsnips, radishes,
rutabagas, salsify, sauerkraut, spinach,
squash, swiss chard, tomatoes, turnips,
watercress

Beneficial Combination

all whole cereal grains, breakfast foods,
bread, cake, candy, chestnuts, cookies,
macaroni, refined rice, spaghetti,
tapioca, sugar, syrup

Carbohydrates
(starch & sugar)

Detrimental Combination

Detrimental Combination

Fruits

Proteins

Food Combining Chart by Theodore A. Baroody, Jr., MA-DC.

OILS

Acid -- All animal fats.
Alkaline -- Corn, olive, canola.
Neutral -- Almond, avocado, butter, coconut, cream, margarine, safflower, sesame, soy, sunflower.

SUGARS

Acid -- Brown, cane, malt, maple syrup, milk, molasses, powdered, white.
Alkaline -- Honey

MISCELLANEOUS FOODS & BEVERAGES

Acid -- Alcoholic beverages, coffee, coffee substitutes, caffeine drinks, drugs, gelatins, mate, nutritional yeast, soy sauce, tobacco, all refined and processed foods.
Alkaline -- Agar agar, brewer's yeast, miso, seaweeds
Alkaline Teas -- Alfalfa, clover, mint, sage, strawberry.

PHYSIOLOGY OF FOOD COMBINING

STARCHES AND VEGETABLES -- Starch digests in the mouth by the action of ptyalin, an enzyme in our saliva.

Starches combine excellently with vegetables but not with proteins. When protein starts digesting, hydrochloric acid is secreted in the stomach to aid digestion. Starches don't do well in this acid medium. They just stop digesting. In fact, the starch neutralizes the acid, so protein digestion slows considerably. The result is a process called <u>putrefaction</u>, in which a climate for toxins and illness is created because these starches and proteins are sitting in the stomach and intestines and not being digested properly.

PROTEIN -- Improper digestion is much like mashing your meat and potatoes together on a plate and just letting them sit there in the open for days. You can imagine what happens. Something similar happens in your body. I advise you to eat only one high-protein food at a meal. If two different high-protein foods like milk and meat are eaten together, the amounts of digestive secretions for milk may stop the digestive action of the meat. Then <u>both</u> proteins would be incompletely digested. Proteins combine best with non-starchy vegetables

125

and succulent vegetables.

A curious thing happens if you eat proteins (except nuts and cheeses) with citrus or other acid foods. Since it takes acid to help digest protein (meats, fish, etc.) you would think citrus, being acid, would help. What actually happens is that citrus acids become alkaline-forming in the stomach and inhibits the secretion of the gastric juices necessary for the digestion of proteins. For instance, if you put vinegar on your salad and eat a protein meal with it, these acids will become alkaline in the stomach and inhibit the production of hydrochloric acid!

Nuts and cheeses are an exception. These can be combined with these acidic citrus fruits. This is because the high fat content of nuts and cheeses will postpone gastric secretions until the citrus is assimilated.

FRUITS -- Now here is one nobody wants to hear, especially HHS sufferers. It is important to know, because this combination is often a cause of HHS irritation and ascending of the stomach. If you put sweet fruits like figs, raisins, sweet grapes, bananas, dates or prunes together with starches such as breads, they will ferment in the stomach. This occurs because the mouth doesn't secrete ptyalin when sugar is present. Starch needs salivary ptyalin to begin its breakdown. If you put starches such as red and sweet fruits together in your mouth, the starch won't get ptyalin, because the sugar won't let it secrete. This means that starch digestion does not occur in the mouth, so the starch then delays the sugars and/or sweet fruits in the stomach, causing fermentation. Examples of this poor combination include: date, raisin and prune bread. Don't get discouraged! There's still plenty to eat in the right combinations. I just want to help you keep that HHS down!

It is recommended to eat melons alone. This is because they digest quickly in the intestines. If they are held up in the stomach by other foods, they quickly decompose and ferment. For HHS sufferers, it is very good to make a meal of a melon. Berries and other fresh fruits may be combined with melons safely.

FAT -- Don't eat too much fat. What happens is that fat lessens the activity of gastric secretions up to 50%. Fat also insulates food particles with a protective fatty shield, so they don't get digested as well. We do have a lifesaver here, though -- green vegetables, especially raw. These wonderful plants will counteract the effect of fat. If you eat a fat-protein meal, eat plenty of fresh, raw, green vegetables with it.

MILK - Drink milk alone, if at all! Its high protein and fat content stimulates the enzymes pepsin and renin to coagulate the milk in the stomach. This causes quite a problem, because the other foods you may eat with milk, like grains, cereals or starches, are prevented from digestion. This happens because the coagulated milk particles cling to the other foods and insulate them from the necessary gastric juices by sheer interference! HHS sufferers beware! This causes the whole mess to putrefy; however, milk does somewhat combine with acid fruits. Examples of these are currants, oranges, pineapples, grapefruits, strawberries, and tangerines.

I especially do not recommend the consumption of pasteurized milk. There are volumes written on this subject. I may add that many allergies are promoted, as well as mucous-producing illnesses. If you feel you must drink milk, try to obtain unpasteurized raw milks, especially goat's milk.

HIATAL HERNIA SYNDROME DIET

*After HHS symptoms have been reduced or disappeared, it is
absolutely essential that you stay with a suitable diet.
Plan to follow this program for at least two years if you expect
lasting results.*

Two different diets are included. The first is based on low blood sugar approaches with some alterations to consider the HHS. Although the second diet is more stringent, it produces excellent results.

Before breakfast: A small bowl of yogurt or one-half
grapefruit.

At breakfast: Take 1 or 2 tablets of betaine HCL and pepsin
then eat: 1 or 2 eggs, or 1 slice of whole wheat bread. It
may be toasted with plenty of butter. Herb teas or coffee
substitutes like Cafix or Pero.

2 Hours after breakfast: A snack of 2 shrimp, or raw nuts, raisins and seeds.

At lunch: Salad (large serving of lettuce, tomato, vinegar or lemon and oil dressing). Vegetables if desired. One-half slice of bread or toast only, with plenty of butter. Dessert: See below list of allowable foods. Beverage

2 hours after lunch: Nuts (almonds), raisins, seeds (sunflower), OR piece of fruit.

2 hours before dinner: Light snack of raw nuts, cheese or celery stuffed with cheese.

At dinner: Take 1 or 2 tablets of betaine HCL and pepsin then eat: Soup if desired (not thickened with flour), vegetables, liberal portion of fish or poultry, beverage

2 hours after dinner: Dessert: an unsweetened gelatin with homemade whipped cream (no sugar). May sweeten with maple syrup or honey OR, fruit from one of the allowables listed below.

Every 2 hrs. until bedtime: A small handful of nuts, raisins, and seeds.

Allowed Vegetables: Asparagus, avocados, beets, broccoli, brussel sprouts, cabbage, cauliflower, carrots, celery, cucumbers, egg plant, onions, peas, radishes, sauerkraut, squash, string beans, tomatoes, turnips, unpeeled potatoes. Lettuce (preferably leaf, or Romaine, avoid iceberg), mushrooms, raw nuts, and brown rice may be taken as freely as desired.

Allowed Fruits: Fresh apples, grapes, plums, peaches, bananas, grapefruit, pineapple, etc. If on occasion you feel you must use some canned fruits, be sure they are unsweetened. These may be cooked or raw, with or without cream, but definitely no sugar.

Allowed Juices: Any unsweetened fruit juice: cranberry, apple, or vegetable juice is allowable.

Allowed Beverages: Herb teas and coffee substitutes. Once on the road to recovery you may sweeten your drinks with Tupelo honey if desired. Remember, use honey only in mild cases or after the initial program is relaxed.

Allowed Desserts: Unsweetened gelatins.

Avoid these foods: Alcoholic beverages such as wine, beer, whiskey, and mixed drinks. Avoid all soft drinks, sugars, candy, cake, pie, pudding and ice cream, caffeine, ordinary coffee, strongly brewed tea, spaghetti, macaroni, noodles, donuts, jams, and jellies.

ALTERNATIVE DIET TO HELP THE H.H.S.

1. *Begin by eating less:*
Meat
Dairy products
Wheat
Eggs
Eliminate all refined sugars and processed foods because these foods form mucous in the system. This mucous interferes with cellular function and increases the amount of protein acid waste products in the tissues.

2. *Eat 60% to 75% of your foods fresh and raw*. Maintain the alkaline-acid ratio of 80% alkaline to 20% acid forming foods with each meal.

3. *Do not begin this diet all at once*. Take your time and slowly move into more fresh foods and less of the meats, wheat, eggs and dairy. Take as much time as you need.

Sample Menu:
Breakfast: Fresh fruits, juice and/or herb tea.
Snack: Raw nuts, raisins, seeds or more fruit.
Lunch: Large salad with sprouts, and dressing.
Dinner: Lightly steamed vegetables, small portion of chicken or fish, (until completely eliminated from diet), tossed salad, or beans and rice and tossed salad.

This is only a sample. There are many ways to prepare vegetables and fruits as main courses and still get the protein and bulk that is desired.

I am often asked, "What is the absolute <u>best</u> dietary recommendation to help my Hiatal Hernia Syndrome?" My answer invariably is, "**Undereat**." Eat only when your stomach feels true hunger pangs. Do not eat just to eat. When your true hunger pangs cease, *stop eating!* Following this one suggestion will make you feel better and reduce the recurrence of HHS symptoms.

Chapter 35

WHAT CAN BE DONE?

Help! How does one stop this "Insidious Syndrome?"

In most cases help begins as a control measure. It seems that the Hiatal Hernia Syndrome (HHS) may recur, even after your most persistent corrections. *Do not* be discouraged. *Do not* give up and throw in the towel. The reason one of the things I call this problem is the "insidious link" is because it is insidious in more than just diagnosis and correction. It is insidious by recurrence. If the stomach can be kept in place for 4 to 6 months and proper measures taken to maintain correction by continued diet and one or more of the exercises given in this book, there is definite hope for long-term repair of the damaged diaphragmatic muscle.

Diagram #15

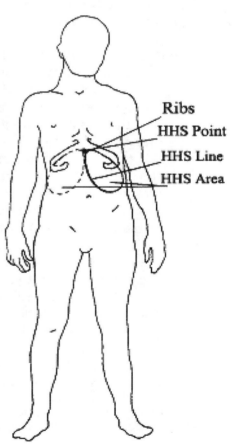

Ribs

HHS Point

HHS Line

HHS Area

ANATOMY

I am devising some new terms to better understand how to check for the HHS, where to correct it, and how to correct it.

In Diagram #15, there is a picture of the left lower ribs and stomach area. The point at the bottom of the breastbone is called the "HHS point."
Next, the line marked along the bottom of the left ribs is called

the "HHS line."

Third is the "HHS area." It is the area about a hand's width across, below the "HHS point" and line on the left side.

Keep these three new areas in mind and refer to the diagrams as needed in order to check and correct the HHS.

HOW TO CHECK THE STOMACH TO DETERMINE IF THE HHS IS PRESENT:

For purposes of a conclusive check, it is necessary to have assistance.

I suggest that a *45-degree slant board* be acquired or constructed in order to give the patient and one who may be helping a much easier angle from which to work. The pictures in this book are taken with the person on a flat surface. Despite the fact that a slanted table would be better for testing and correction, after 25 years of working on the HHS, almost no one has such a table. I do not expect the public to use one unless the reader is fortunate enough to make one.

INSTRUCTIONS FOR THE ASSISTANT: (FRIEND OR PHYSICIAN)

1. Place the patient on the slant board or flat table, head at top. This can be done on the floor. Put a pillow under the person's head.
2. Ask the person to breathe one time as deeply as he can and just observe. He should be able to inhale down to the pubic area. If he can't, the HHS may be present.
3. Next, have the person raise and lock one arm with a straightened elbow. (See Photo #1.) Ask him to try to stop you as you pull down on the straightened arm. The arm should hold firmly. Move easily into the muscle test. Do not suddenly try to jerk the arm down. Make sure the client knows you are ready to start by saying "Ready, resist." Put your fingers on the "HHS point" (Use oil). (See Photo #2.) Ask that he breathe in and out. Then ask him to hold his breath out while you stroke the "HHS line" quickly and firmly with your fingers. (See Photo #3.) Ask that he try to stop you again as you pull down on the straightened arm. If the arm goes weak, the HHS is present. (See Photo #4.)

(Note: If you must attempt to check without assistance, touch the "HHS point" and stroke the "HHS line." Almost invariably when the HHS is present, you will feel pain or tightness, sometimes all the way through to the back.)

Photo #1

Photo #2

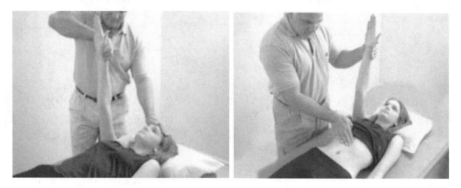

Photo #3

Photo #4

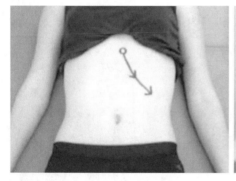
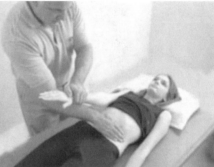

HHS Point And Line

**Hand Moves Along HHS Line
Then Arm Is Tested For Weakness**

HOW TO CORRECT THE H.H.S.

This technique is not difficult. Be assured, you can do it.

1. Start by putting your hands, one on top of the other, on the "HHS area" so that your fingertips touch the "HHS point." (See Diagram #16.)

2. Pull firmly with your fingers and fingertips downwards over the "HHS line." (See Photos #4A & #4B & Diagram #16.)

133

Photo #4A   Photo #4B

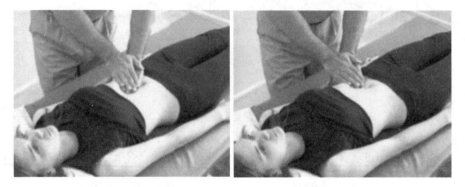

Diagram #16

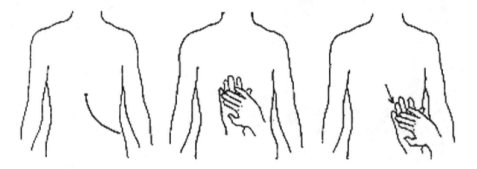

3. Repeat. (Usually it takes at least 8 to 10 good tugs and with some people closer to 25 tugs is required.)

4. During the process you may hear the stomach gurgle. This means it is starting to move down. Keep tugging until you feel the stomach has done all the moving it is going to do at the time. People differ on this. Some stomachs make no sound as they slip back into place.

5. Now to check if the HHS is corrected, repeat step #3 in "How to Check for the HHS". Pull firmly on the left "HHS area" with your fingers while asking the person to exhale. Then, ask him to raise his arm and resist you with all his strength and see if his arm is stronger. (See Photo #1.)

6.   Ask the person to inhale deeply. If he can breathe to the pubic area, the HHS is corrected. If he can't inhale this far, more than likely the stomach is blocking the lungs' ability to do so. In other words, the HHS is still present! If so, keep trying. Sometimes the stomach is very stubborn, and other techniques given later must be employed in conjunction with this one. You can be absolutely sure the HHS is corrected if the arm stays strong and breathing is deep. The key words to ask after treatment are: "Do you feel longer, looser and lighter in the stomach area?" He will usually report one or all of these.

HOW TO CORRECT THE H.H.S. IN CHILDREN

Use the same technique as above; however, instead of using your whole hand, use only one or two fingers. The main thing to remember with children is to take it slowly and be gentle. The HHS will correct very easily in most of these cases.

WHAT MAY BE EXPERIENCED AS THE STOMACH IS CORRECTED

Many times, if the stomach has been especially high in the diaphragm, relief may be expressed in several different ways:

1.   Don't be surprised if you belch after the stomach is down. Sometimes this will go on for quite a while. Don't worry; it is normal. This is allowing excessive air to come out of the trapped upper stomach area.

2.   Don't be surprised if you feel like crying after the HHS is corrected. The body is under such stress in this area that crying is a blessed relief and allows the diaphragm to relax. You might say these are "tears of joy."

3.   The ability to breathe deeply will be experienced. Breathe all the way down to the lower abdomen. (See Diagram #17.)

Diagram #17

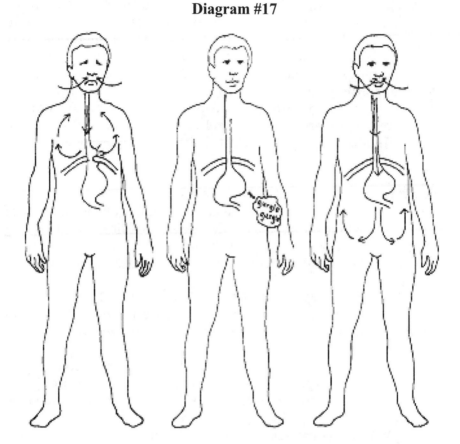

4. Shakiness can occur because when the HHS is corrected, the body can express its true need for increased blood sugar. This causes an already stressed system to utilize quickly what little blood sugar is available once the stomach becomes operable; therefore, the body shakes and sometimes becomes cold. It usually takes about fifteen minutes for the body to readjust the blood sugar levels after the HHS is in place. The client may report that they are hungry. This is a good sign that the stomach is synchronizing with the rest of the digestive system.

PRACTICAL APPLICATIONS

This section gives techniques for the times immediate relief is needed, as well as suggestions to keep the stomach down over extended periods so that it may heal itself. Choose those that suit your individual needs. Many may be done in combination with others.

IMMEDIATE ACTION

The person who finds himself in great pain or difficulty but is not able to get outside help must help himself on the spot. The critical need is signaled by these classical symptoms:

1. Moderate to severe pain or discomfort at the "HHS point".
2. An upset, nauseated feeling.
3. Tightness in the chest.
4. Inability to breathe deeply, which feels like choking or smothering.
5. Constant belching, sometimes with reflux.
6. Sour stomach.

SUGGESTIONS FOR RELIEF ARE:

1. *Bouncing* -- In the absence of a serious spinal injury, bouncing is a good exercise. (For persistent cases, bounce as a regular exercise every morning.) (See Diagram #18.)
   a. Drink one or two glasses of water. This provides weight in the stomach.
   b. Bounce 12 times on your heels. Shake the floor! This jarring effect will pull the stomach back down into place. This technique works with gravity very nicely.
   c. Take a deep breath and notice if you can breathe down to your lower abdomen.

Diagram #18

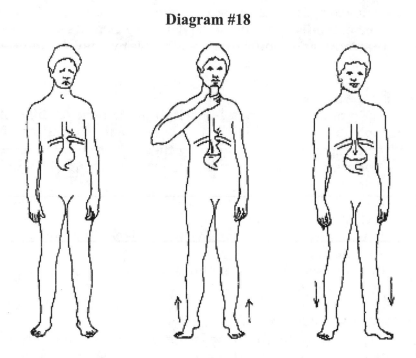

2. *Gentle manipulation of hiatal hernia into place* - Put your hands on the "HHS point" as is shown in Diagram #16. Coordinate your breathing so that you push down firmly on the stomach when you are exhaling. By the time you reach the navel area, you should have exhaled completely. Repeat this several times until you feel longer, looser, or lighter in the area. You may hear or feel a gurgling as the stomach drops. (See Diagram #16.)

3. *Leg Cross* - Lie on your left side and put the right leg out over the left leg. (See Photo #5.) This might be done on a couch or off the side of a bed or table. Hold this position for about one minute. This will sometimes release the HHS.

Photo #5

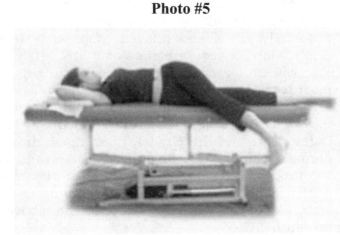

4. *Hand Warmth* -- To help yourself or others, one of the most effective methods is simply laying the hands on the stomach area directly on the "HHS point" and "HHS area." (See Diagram #19.) This is especially good and recommended for the elderly. It seems that the warmth

Diagram #19

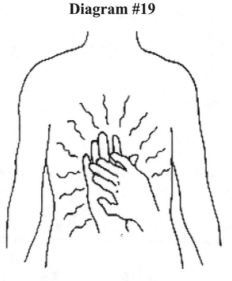

generated by the hands has a wonderfully relaxing effect on the diaphragm and other stomach muscles. This allows the stomach to drop down. You may hear the

139

gurgling sound here. This is one of the procedures I highly recommend. It may take longer, however, so plan to spend at least 10 minutes with the hands in place. In my experience, it is often better during this time to be absolutely silent and relaxed. If possible use the 45-degree slant board, but this is not absolutely necessary. You will find correction of the HHS in this manner a most rewarding experience.

5. *Trigger Points* -- There is a trigger-point on the head for the vagus nerve. (See Diagram #20.) Use it to relax the vagus nerve and thereby let the stomach drop back into normal position. Use fingertip pressure and hold for 7 seconds; releases then repeat two more times. Trigger points for the stomach are also found on the hand and foot. (See Diagram #20.) Repeat the above fingertip pressure procedure.

Diagram #20

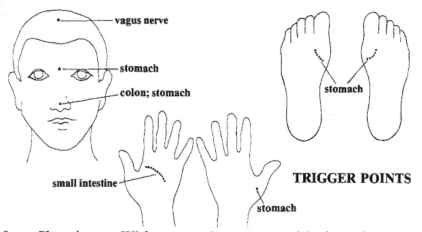

TRIGGER POINTS

6. *Slapping* -- With an assistant, try this but do it with some caution and not too hard. While standing, have someone gently slap the area below the throat and simultaneously have him gently slap the opposite side on the back. (See Photos #6 & #7.) Do this about 6 times. On occasion this will free the stomach to drop into place.

(Do not do this if there are heart complications or a pacemaker.)

Photo #6   Photo #7

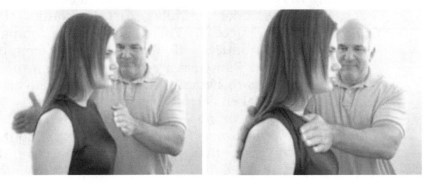

The preceding techniques are suitable even in work situations - construction, factory, and office, and can be done in conjunction with the daily prevention techniques and diet.

EVERYDAY PREVENTION

Everyday prevention consists of many techniques to keep the stomach down when you aren't necessarily in pain and to strengthen the stomach area.

1. *Consistent maintenance of good posture* will allow less crowding in the abdominal area which is conducive to keeping the stomach in proper location.
2. *Do not overeat!* Eat light meals about 6 to 8 times a day. Follow the diet suggestions in the "HHS and Diet" chapter.
3. *Chew your food very thoroughly, at least 25 times per mouthful.*
4. *It is well always to eat in a harmonious atmosphere.* The best music for the digestive system is Mozart.
5. *Drink liquid between meals, rather than with meals.* Liquid dilutes hydrochloric acid, thereby reducing the stomach's ability to digest food.
6. *Digestive aids* -- The use of H.H.S. Formula and Pan-Gest has been very successful over many years with thousands of people. These formulas stimulate HCL production as opposed to adding more. If you find that more HCL support is definitely needed, then betaine hydrochloride is recommended instead. Formulas

containing pancreatin, comfrey, papaya, and ox bile extract work well. Pan-Gest contains many different food enzymes including protease, amylase and lipase. You can also take formulas just containing these enzymes with success. There are many companies selling good products. If these enzyme containing formulas such as Pan-Gest are taken with the meal, and you still need more betaine HCL support, then betaine HCL should be taken 30 minutes after eating.

7.   *Inhale through your nose and pull the air all the way down to the pubic area.* Exhale through your mouth as much as you can; then, repeat this procedure three times. If you get a little lightheaded, it will go away quickly.

8.   *Dr. Robert Down's Original Formula:* 1 part Aloe Vera juice and 1 part papaya juice mixed 50/50 with sugar-free ginger ale or club soda. Sip all through the day. Do not gulp! This is a winner; it really helps.

9.   *Do not consume ice cold foods or liquids,* as these can definitely shock the system and cause the stomach to ascend. This is especially true if the HHS is already a problem for you.

10.   *Use ginger root extract.* This may be purchased or made the following way: Squeeze the fresh ginger root until you get juice. A juicer is preferable here. Take one teaspoon every morning on an empty stomach. Do this daily until the stomach is better, at least one month. Repeat in the future if the stomach starts going up again. Many have reported this to be a miracle cure for the hiatal hernia syndrome.

11.   *Use Swedish Bitters* (sold at most health food stores) as directed on the bottle. This formulation has been shown throughout the years to safely aid digestion.

LONG-TERM ONGOING PREVENTION

Long-term prevention means just that. Many readers will have had the HHS for many years.

1.   *Avoid heavy lifting and improper lifting* (see Diagram #21). They are major causes of the HHS. If you don't breathe out when you lift, it will force the stomach into the esophagus.

Diagram #21

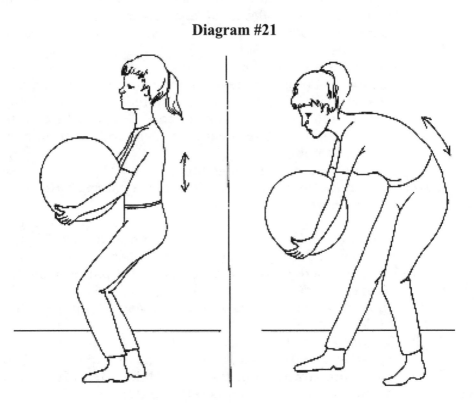

2.   *Avoid overly strenuous exercise in which the abdominal muscles are used.*

3.   *Do not swallow air.* This is a nervous habit, which seems to aggravate the HHS. The habit results from hunger and anxiety produced when the HHS presses against the lungs. It induces acidosis to a mild degree. If you catch yourself doing this, breathe as deeply as you can. Yawning is a mechanism that will relax the diaphragm and allow deeper breathing. You may even hear your stomach gurgle a bit as it drops down.

4.   *Swimming.* This is a most beneficial exercise, as it strengthens and relaxes the diaphragm at the same time. Water is a very relaxing medium for all kinds of stress.

5.   *Elevate the posts at the head of the bed between 3 inches and 6 inches, or sleep on a wedge pillow.* This will keep your head higher than your stomach. Many HHS problems are much worse at night.

6. *Have a massage to the stomach and the small intestine area done by a professional massage therapist.*
7. *Avoid tight clothing, especially around the stomach area.*
8. *Take Epsom salts baths, approximately three cups per tub, and pull the stomach down while soaking.* Also, whirlpool, sauna, or steam baths will help the stomach area to relax. Try massaging the stomach while engaging in these relaxing aids. How often? Gauge according to your stress level. Use the stress scale and determine by number of points.
9. *Pull-ups or just hanging by hands.*
10. *Using door frame, hands braced above, swing forward to loosen rib cage.*
11. *Drink slippery elm tea.* Steep 5 minutes, serve at room temperature, <u>not</u> <u>hot</u>. This will help to soothe the stomach and prepare the way for digestion. Especially recommended for those who have the paraesophageal hernia.
12. *Drink valerian root tea to relax.* Steep 5 minutes and drink heated.
13. *Centaury is an herb long renowned for its abilities to help digestive disturbances.* I have found it quite useful in herbal preparations for the HHS. Make a tea with it and sweeten with honey as it is rather bitter.
14. *The homeopathic formula, Lycopodium is good for H.H.S.*
15. *Vagus nerve exercises*: These will relax the vagus and sometimes drop the stomach into place. Sit with spine erect, body relaxed, inhale through nostrils deeply. Hold your breath and roll head from left to right, making a complete circle. Relax the neck muscles while doing this. Start with 5 times and gradually end with 30 times. Now do the reverse. Inhale, hold your breath and roll your head from right to left. Repeat the same number of times in each direction.
16. *Avoid coughing if you definitely have the HHS. Coughing can aggravate it.*
17. *Avoid sneezing.*
18. *Stress control techniques:*
    a. Breath control -- One of the best ways to control stress is controlled breathing. By slowing the heart beat down, you can control "flight or fight" response that stress induces. Teach yourself to

pause for two seconds between normal breaths. Most people find that when they control their breathing in this way, their heart rate drops 5 or even 10 beats below normal. Your heart is being given a chance to relax because you are putting less demand on it to circulate the oxygen to your body.

b. Muscle relaxation -- Stress and tension have come to mean almost the same thing because most Americans have developed terrible muscle-tensing habits whenever they feel a little stressed. This exercise may help. It comes from yoga relaxation postures and has been adapted here: Lie on your back. Starting with the feet, contract all the muscles in toes, feet, ankles so that they scrunch together. Hold the contraction for several seconds; then let all those muscles relax as completely as you can. Pause and think about the relaxation in your feet. Then, contract the calf muscles. Hold the tension there briefly; then relax. Now put the tension into your thigh muscles; hold then relax. Pause and think about the feeling you now have throughout the legs. To complete this exercise, simply repeat the tensing-relaxing pattern throughout the rest of the body. From legs to abdomen, lower back, chest upper back, shoulders, hands, forearms, and upper arms, neck, jaw muscles and at last, your face. With daily practice, this can be the most effective way to release tension from the large muscles. It's great to do right before you go to sleep and right after you wake up.

c. Quiet time -- Sit quietly for a few moments each day. To focus or center yourself, direct your attention to your heartbeat or breath, so you can tune out all the outer activity. Perhaps you may want to chant a word (silently or out loud). The repetition of uplifting words is greatly relaxing, but is not absolutely necessary. You may choose to say a quiet prayer.

19. *Spinal pressure technique.* When the stomach just doesn't seem to want to drop into place, try this

technique: Start by getting a friend to locate the important pressure points. Usually one or all of these points are quite tender on one side of the spine or the other. Have your friend use his thumb on the most tender spots. Hold for seven seconds, then release. Do this two more times on each sore spot, a total of three times at seven seconds each time. You may wonder how hard to press. The idea is not to inflict unnecessary amounts of pain; however, it must be firm enough to relieve the pain. Also, be sure to press either side of the vertebrae that are painful or tender. Amazingly, the involvement may reduce considerably, just by using the thumb on these points. This technique alone may help the stomach to release and relieve pain and anxiety. (If you feel reluctant to do this, let a chiropractor or osteopath work on these areas for you.)

a.   The first point is called D-4. To find it start at the bottom of the neck and find the most prominent vertebrae sticking out. It will feel like a big bony knob. (See Diagram #10) The others will not be as prominent. D-4 is the fifth bony knob (vertebrae) down. This is the main one for most people, because it relates to the sliding type of hiatal hernia which is 90% of most problems.

b.   Next, go down two more bony knobs. This is D-6. It may be sore also. Repeat the same procedure as before. Press three times for seven seconds.

c.   Keep counting down from D-6 three more knobs to D-9. Repeat procedure. Finally, go down one more knob to D-10 and press on the left side. One or more of these points will be sensitive.

20. *The HHS Stomach Egg.* After 20 plus years of giving people instructions on how to work on their Hiatal Hernia Syndrome for themselves, I think I have found a better answer. Some people report that it is too painful on their hands to do the HHS maneuver as I have described it, because of individual hand problems. Others say that they find it hard to do but do it anyway because it helps them enormously. Some years ago I started out with an engineer, designing a tool made out of plastic or rubber that might help push the stomach down. The only workable thing we could come up with

146

was very expensive and difficult to make. In frustration I said to my engineer friend, "Andy, what I need is something more basic, simpler. Surely God won't let this problem go unresolved with so many hurting people out there calling me every day and depending on me for answers. The thing I am looking for is something like this odd sized egg here on Wanda's craft table." I picked it up and positioned the egg under my ribs and pushed. It was a perfect fit and eliminated all the discomfort of using your own hands to pull down the hiatal hernia, and to stop its devastating group of painful symptoms. The egg did it better!

Oh, yes, by the way, I made this little discovery on Easter Day. It seems God does have a sense of humor.

Photo #8

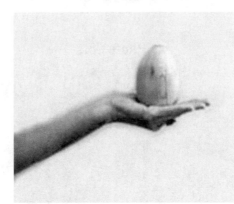

Photo #8A

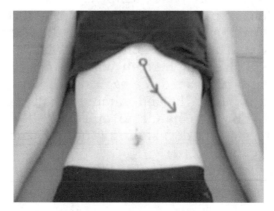

**HHS Beginning Point And Line To Follow
When Making HHS Correction**

Photo #8B

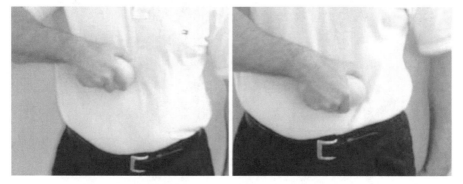

**Method To Work On HHS With The Egg Or Hands
(Can Be Done Standing Or Lying Down)**

Many times correction of the H.H.S. alone is not sufficient. After many years of experimentation, I have developed muscle checks for a "stuck diaphragm". A stuck diaphragm creates pain in the chest and shortness of breath. If these symptoms do not subside after have done the H.H.S. maneuvers, suspect a stuck diaphragm.

I am giving two methods of checking for this and four methods for rebalancing it. Usually, one of these rebalancing measures works for everyone. From what I have ascertained, it is the major blood vessels going through the diaphragm that seem to get "stuck." This restricts the movement of the diaphragm and refers pain viscerally to the chest and structurally to anywhere from C4 in the neck to T12, which is in the mid-lower back. Occasionally rib pains (which sometimes feel like they are broken) are the result of this misalignment.

MUSCLE CHECK NO. 1 FOR A "STUCK" DIAPHRAGM BECAUSE OF ABDOMINAL AORTA:
1. Person is standing extending arms straight out and to the sides. (See Photo #9.)
2. Tester puts knee in stomach and attempts to pull both arms forward at the same time. (See Photo #10.) A weakness indicates a problem with the diaphragm.

Photo #9   **Photo #10**

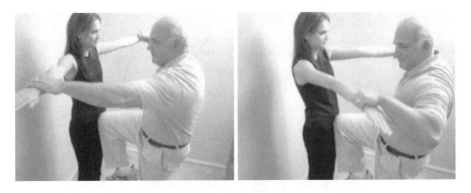

MUSCLE CHECK NO. 2 FOR A "STUCK" DIAPHRAGM BECAUSE OF INFERIOR VENA CAVA:
1. Person is standing extending arms straight out and to the sides. (See photos #11 & #12.)
2. Tester puts knee in back and attempts to pull both arms backward at the same time. A weakness indicates a stuck diaphragm.

Photo #11   **Photo #12**

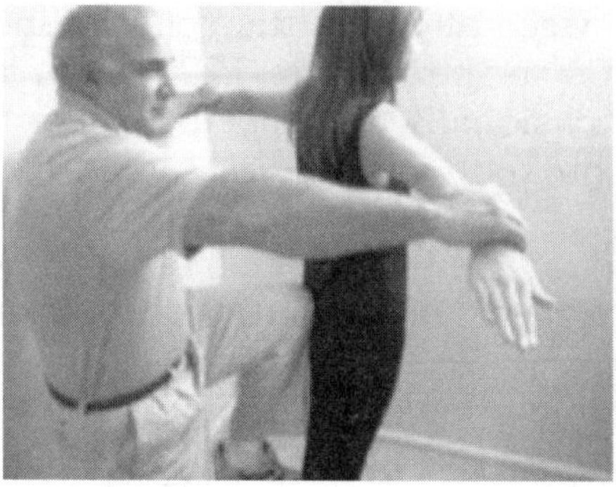

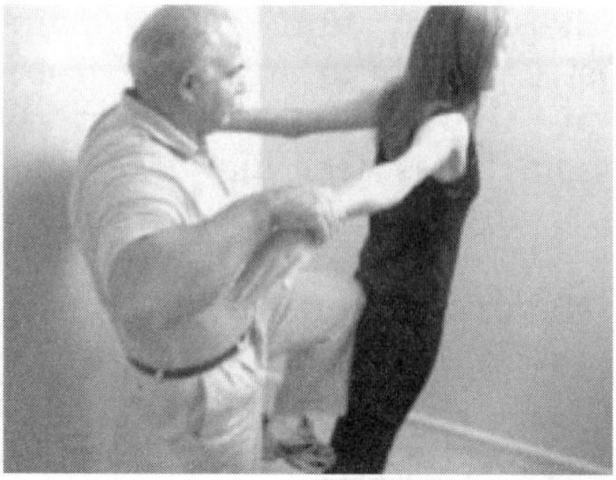

THE METHODS OF CORRECTION FOLLOW:

FIRST METHOD:

1. Person stands back to back with tester and locks both arms.
2. Tester lifts person slightly off ground by bending forward. (See Photo #13.)

NOTE: Only do this if no other structural problems will be made worse by doing so. This is my preferred method of rebalancing this problem. Use your common sense.

Photo #13

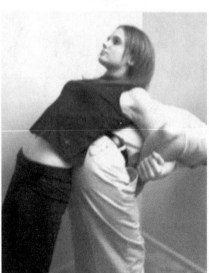

SECOND METHOD:

1. Person is lying down on back. Have them exhale, pushing the stomach toward the spine.
2. Tester puts hands under rib cage as diagram shows, attempting to stretch the muscle. This will help to free the vessels. (See Photo #14.)

Photo #14

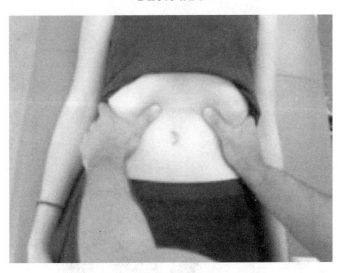

Third Method:

1. Person is lying down on back.
2. Tester puts fingers two inches over and one inch down from both sides of the navel and pushes inward, holding for a count of ten. (See Photo #15.)

    NOTE: This can be uncomfortable. Go slowly into the points.

Photo #15

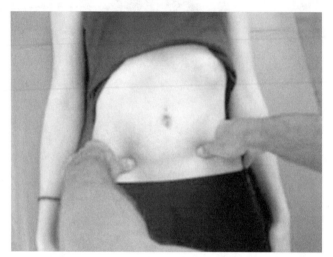

Fourth Method:
1. Person is on back.
2. Tester locates a point over the femur heads and presses inward for a count of ten. (See Photo #16.)

NOTE: These last two methods are diaphragm reflex points discovered in clinical situations to be helpful with a "stuck" diaphragm.

Photo #16

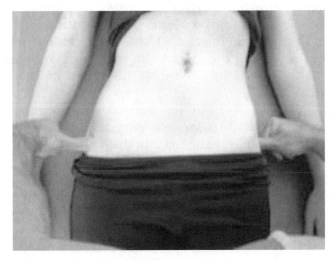

The need for digestive enzymes warrants repetition here. These can be purchased at natural food stores and sometimes in the vitamin sections of grocery stores, drug stores, or from your health practitioner. For betaine hydrochloride users it is difficult to prescribe the exact number of pills to take per meal. A general rule is to start with one per meal, five minutes before you eat and increase this amount by one per day, per meal, until you notice a slight burning discomfort in the stomach. When this occurs take ¼ teaspoon of baking soda in 4 ounces of water. This will neutralize the excess betaine HCL. Then back down one pill per meal to the point that it does not burn. This will be the proper dosage. For example, let's say you were up to three per meal and the burning started. You back down to two per meal and stay there. Because it is recommended that you eat smaller meals and more regularly so the food will assimilate better, I still only recommend the betaine hydrochloride to be taken with the three major meals. *It is definitely not recommended to take betaine hydrochloride if there is an active ulcer.*

To help with the H.H.S. and all aspects of digestion, I formulated the supplement, H.H.S. Formula. It has performed beyond all my expectations to naturally alleviate the symptoms this difficult and dangerous syndrome. It is a very balanced food supplement that has resulted in the alleviation of HHS symptoms for thousands of people over the last 15 years, and that is why I recommend it throughout the book.

Pan-Gest was formulated to assist in every part of the digestive cycle. It is for problems with bloating, indigestion, gall bladder, pancreas, liver, and small intestines imbalances in particular. Anything that has to do with the pancreas will be addressed with Pan-Gest including all types of blood sugar imbalances.

Glyco-Well was formulated to help with the more serious forms of blood sugar imbalances, particularly hyperglycemia. After the HHS has taken its toll on the body for so long, low blood sugar gives way to high blood sugar (diabetes). Glyco-Well is a natural preventative. It is in no way a substitute for any medication. It assists with the various functions of the pancreas and liver to support their balance. In doing so, the ravages of blood sugar imbalances can be lessened. Again, this is not a drug and should not be considered as one. It is only a therapeutic food supplement which supports the body in certain ways.

INSTANCES WHEN PROFESSIONALS ARE NEEDED

As a professional-osteopath, chiropractor, or naturopath, you have experience in diagnosing and correcting spinal misalignments. From my accumulated clinical experience and the piece-by-piece references of many other health authorities concerning the hiatal hernia, I present an organized approach to help control this problem for your patients.

Don't get discouraged if they do not respond immediately or only respond for a very short period of time. The odds are in your favor. Keep encouraging your patients; eventually, the HHS will stabilize. Of course continued care may be necessary after stabilization in order for the damaged diaphragm to heal. Remember, if you can free the stomach and, more importantly, the vagus nerve branch into the stomach for even a short period of time, you have increased your patient's ability to function, digest, assimilate, eliminate, and enjoy being pain free.

The HHS can be very tricky. Another name I have for it is "the great trickster", because one year I missed it in fourteen of my most difficult cases. The clients were not improving, regardless of what I did. (I have a lot of rabbits in my hat!) The symptoms were so deceiving that even I, who have trained myself to be on constant alert for this syndrome, was misled.

Only after completely rethinking the situations did I conclude that "the insidious link" had to be involved, even though my kinesiological tests did not find it. I manually adjusted the stomach on each of these patients anyway. To my surprise, each of them started making rapid improvement.

The most frequently noted misalignments accompanying the Hiatal Hernia Syndrome (HHS) include:

1. D-4, the fourth dorsal vertebrae on the right side. This is the most common misalignment in the sliding type of HHS.
2. D-6, the sixth dorsal vertebrae on the right side.
3. D-7 thru D-9, the seventh, eighth and ninth dorsal vertebrae on the right side. D-9 is always found in the paraesophageal type of HHS and many times with the sliding type as well. This does not mean that if a D-9 misalignment is present, it is definitely the more serious paraesophageal hernia. The D-9 misalignment is present when the paraesophogeal hernia is present.
4. D-10 will sometimes be tender on the left side.
5. An anterior misalignment of the second rib on the right side.
6. For cranial adjusters: the right temporal bone will be inferior. Usually it is corrected on inhalation.
7. Always palpate and x-ray if suspicious of abdominal aneurysms; however, be aware that only about 2% of the patients you see will have them. Don't be shy about going ahead, if it satisfies your clinical judgment.

For the particularly tough patient, Dr. Failor recommends an interesting technique: Correct the HHS, as is indicated by pulling it down. Use a cotton ball. Compact it to half the size of your fist. Tape it at the "HHS point" with hypoallergenic tape. Leave it, except to bathe, for several days to see if this helps keep the stomach in place. An option to using the tape is to use a rib brace to hold the cotton firmly at the "HHS point."

Chapter 36

EXERCISES FOR THE HHS

These exercises are some of the ones I find that will help to strengthen the diaphragm and allow the HHS not to ride upward. They can assist in an immediate realignment, which can allow for the dropping of the stomach enough to eliminate the pressure being placed on the vagus nerve. If any of these exercises make you feel uncomfortable, select the most appropriate ones to meet your needs.

1. Lie on your back on a flat surface. Extend the legs and raise them until the upper abdomen tightens. With legs still in the air about 12 inches from the floor, separate the legs. Move them back together. Then lower them to the floor. (See Photos #17 & #18.) Do these exercises slowly and only a few times a day until you are able to do more. This strengthens the stomach muscles and the diaphragm.

Photo #17

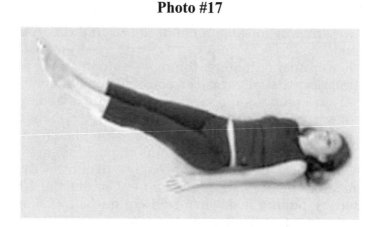

Photo #18

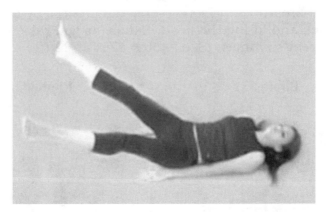

2. Sit in a chair that has arms. Brace your forearms on the arms of the chair. (You can also use a flat bottom chair to hold on to.) Keep the knees together; raise them as far as you can. Inhale as the knees are brought up; then exhale as the knees are brought down. (See Photos #19 & #20.)

Photo #19   **Photo #20**

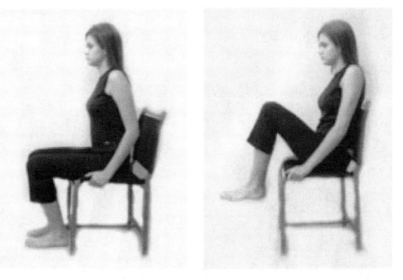

3. Kneel in a "donkey" position, arms and thighs at right angles to the body, spine straight. Bend the head down; at the same time round the spine by humping the back and breathe in. Then reverse the process by arching the back and lifting the head. Exhale as you raise the head. Repeat six times. (See Photos #21 & #22.)

Photo #21   **Photo #22**

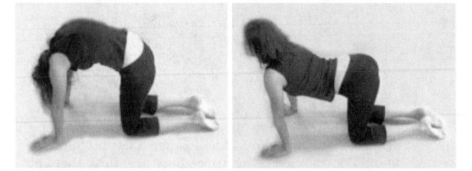

4. Stretch back before and after every meal. You can do this sitting or standing. This lengthens the stomach area and will help to keep it down. If you will notice, animals often do this. Unlike man, animals will also rest after meals to assist digestion. (See Photos #23, #24.)

Photo #23   **Photo #24**

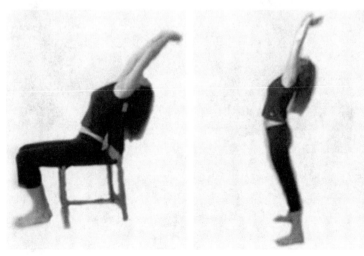

5. This is where the tougher exercises start. They really help but do them only if your body is capable of getting into these positions without additional distress.

6. Sit on your knees, feet tucked back, and toes straight. (Refer to Photos #25 and 26.) Now put your arms out straight and start to lean back. To begin with, you may need the help of another with this one for some time before attempting it on your own. Eventually, even the stiffest of spines will become more flexible. This exercise will definitely help to stabilize the stomach and diaphragm area. Do it daily!

Photo #25   **Photo #26**

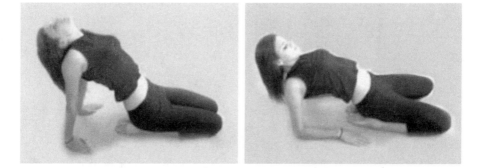

7. This exercise is called the Modified Cobra. Lie on the stomach. Keep the legs together. Put the hands, palm down, beside your shoulders. Roll the eyes up toward the ceiling and let your head and chest arch back very slowly. (See Photo #27.) Hold this position for a few seconds; then, slowly return to a flat position. It is good for stretching and elongating the muscles which directly affect the positioning of the stomach and help the HHS to stay down. This is my favorite exercise for the HHS.

Photo #27

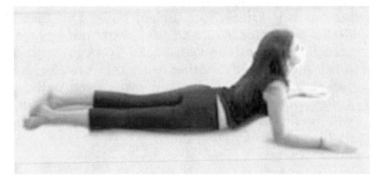

AFTERWORD

In conclusion, I write from the heart. The work I've done on the Hiatal Hernia Syndrome is my contribution to the advancing field of holistic health. Its far-reaching scope surprises even me! It may manifest in an apparently unlimited multitude of ways. I have endeavored to outline only a few. One is amazed and even shocked at the pandemic proportions this unsuspecting problem has taken. Yet, I'm sure there are many symptoms I have yet to discover, as illustrated by the case of Angela. Previously undiscovered compromised biochemical pathways crop up all the time. I appeal to all who would do this work to compile and submit it. If it is found that symptoms are relieved that were heretofore not linked with this syndrome, please let me know. For those who have tried the methods I have recommended and still can find no relief, I would suggest you contact one of our Holographic Health Practitioners. They have been instructed on how to deal with this syndrome and have seen first-hand examples of its deadly effects during their training and later in their offices. There will be many frustrating days as one incorporates this information and gain feeling for it. There still are such days for me. If you have even the least suspicion that this syndrome exists, go with that feeling and start the corrective process. I am asked, "What is the bottom line root cause of the HHS? Why are such an alarmingly high percentage of people afflicted?"

I turn to my feelings and intuition. We are one interconnected species -- plants, animals and man. When a single sparrow falls to the earth on the other side of the planet, each of us knows it. When one person suffers, physically or emotionally, all are affected. Our world is rife with anger at this time. One of every four countries is actually at war. This outer turmoil is felt by everyone -- the harried businessman, and the silent Trappist monk. If we forget our oneness with God, we open our very bodies to this massive assault of dissident feelings.

The sympathetic nervous system is over stimulated, creating systemic tension within our most delicate nerve center -- the solar plexus. This, in turn, tightens the whole of the alimentary (digestive) tract and pulls the stomach upward into an already under-breathing diaphragm. From here, endocrine gland function is immediately lowered because of the strong effects that the HHS seems to have on the thymus gland. Thus, the thymus gland, the immune system regulator, under-functions and leaves us the victim of viral infections and general physiological depletions. This effect returns to increase the HHS, which in turn, perpetuates the impairment of that crucial solar plexus center. The stomach is the hub and point of balance that reflects all the emotions. I rarely find the HHS in one who is truly joyous and happy, for he is balanced within. All foregoing clinical observations such as poor diet, HCL deficiency, inappropriate living habits, long-term systemic stress and vagus nerve disruption only induce physical manifestations of the hernia. It is my conviction that in order to make fundamental corrections of this syndrome, one must love himself for what he is and be at peace with God.

Love is the answer; love oneself; love others.

REFERENCES

Airola, P. Are You Confused? Health Plus Publishers, 1971.
_____ . How to Get Well, Health Plus Publishers, 1974.
_____ . Rejuvenation Secrets from Around the World, Health Plus Publishers, 1974.
_____ . Hypoglycemia: A Better Approach, Health Plus Publishers, 1974.
Anthony, C.A. Basic Concepts in Anatomy & Physiology, C.V. Mosby Co., 1974.
Bailey, J.P., Sensor Perceptor, ES Press, Inc., 1977.
Baker, Jr., C.E., Physician's Desk Reference, Medical Economics Company, Inc., 1984.
Balch, Jr., J.F., Nutritional Outline For the Professional, Balch Publisher, 1983.
Bauam, Stuart. J., Introduction to Organic & Biological Chemistry, MacMillan Publishing Co., Inc., 1978.
Bricklin, M., The Practical Encyclopedia of Natural Healing, Rodale Press, 1983.
Broeringmeyer, R., The Problem Solver Nutritionally Speaking, Creative Printers, 1977.
Campbell, G.W., A Doctor's Proven New Home Cure for Arthritis, Parker Publishing Co., Inc., 1972.
Crook, W., The Yeast Connection, Professional Books, 1983, 1984.
Downs, R. W, Your Grand and Glorious Gastrointestinal System, Bestways Magazine, July 1983.
Faelten, S., The Allergy Self-Help Book, Rodale Press, 1983.
_____ . The Complete Book of Minerals for Health, Rodale Press, 1981.
Failor, R., The New Age Chiropractor, Richard M. Failor Publishers, 1976.
Fincher, J., The Human Body: The Brain, Torstar Books, 1984.
Fredericks, C., Psycho-Nutrition, Grosset & Dunlap Publishers, 1976.
_____ . Look Younger, Feel Healthier, Grosset & Dunlap Publishers, 1977.
Gerras, C., The Complete Book of Vitamins, Rodale Press, 1977.
Guthrie, H.A., Introductory Nutrition, C.V. Mosby Co., 1975.

Guyton, A.C., <u>Basic Human Physiology</u>, W.B. Saunders Co. Publishers, 1977.

Haas, E.M., <u>Staying Healthy With the Seasons</u>, Celestial Arts Publishers, 1981.

Heindel, M., <u>The Mystery of the Ductless Glands</u>, Rosicrucian Fellowship Publishers, 1980.

Holmes, T. and Rahe, R., <u>Social Readjustment Rating Scale</u>, Pergamon Press, 1967.

Jackson, J. & Teague, T., <u>The Handbook of Alternatives to Chemical Medicine</u>, Coconino County, 1975.

Jensen, B., <u>Tissue Cleaning Through Bowel Management</u>, Bernard Jensen, Publisher, 1981.

Jolly, R.T., <u>The Color Atlas of Human Anatomy</u>, Harmony Books, 1980.

Kirshchmann, J.D., <u>Nutrition Almanac</u>, McGraw-Hill, 1979.

Kulvinskas, V., <u>Survival Into the 21st Century</u>, Omangod Press, 1975.

Landau, B., <u>Essential Human Anatomy and Physiology</u>, Scott Foresman & Co., 1980.

Lazarus, R., <u>Psychology, Stress, and the Coping Process</u>, McGraw-Hill, 1971.

McGarey, W.A., <u>Physician's Reference Notebook</u>, A.R.E. Press, 1983.

McMimm, R.M.H. and Hutchings, R.T.: <u>Color Atlas of Human Anatomy</u>, Year Book Medical Publishers, 1977.

Mindell, E., <u>Vitamin Bible</u>, Warner Books, Inc., 1979.

Mullen, P.B., <u>Prescription Drugs</u>, Beekman House, 1985.

Schwartz, E.F., <u>Endocrines, Organs and Their Impact</u>, Edmar Printing, 1979.

Turner, G.D. and St. Clair, M.G.: <u>Individual Reference File</u>, A.R.E. Press, 1976.

Upledger, J.E. and Vredenoogd, J.D., <u>Craniosacral Therapy</u>, Eastland Press, 1983.

Wigmore, A.W., <u>From Fat to Fit</u>, Rising Sun Publications, 1977.

GLOSSARY

Adhesion -- Abnormal fibers which bind organs and tissues to one another, blocking nerve, blood and lymph functions.

Adrenal Glands -- A pair of glands sitting atop the kidneys which produce and secrete many vital hormones.

Bile -- A yellow fluid secreted by the liver into the duodenum. It helps in the digestion and breakdown of fatty foods.

Candida Albicans -- A fungus in the monilia group. It can cause vaginal infections and numerous other conditions, if there is over production in the body.

Cholesterol -- A component of animal oils and fats. It is produced in the liver.

Chyle -- This very important substance is produced in the Peyer's Patches of the small intestine. It coats fat molecules that are transported through the lymph system for energy storage. It is also an alkaline substance which helps to maintain proper acid-alkaline balance.

Chyme -- This is food that has been mixed and acted on by hydrochloric acid and digestive enzymes before it can be passed on to the small intestine.

Diaphragm -- A large dome-shaped muscle which separates the lungs and heart from the stomach, liver, pancreas, kidneys, spleen, small and large intestines. It is the "breathing muscle."

Duodenum -- The first portion of the small intestine, starting after the stomach. It receives bile from the liver, food from the stomach, and enzymes from the pancreas.

Endocrine Glands -- These are glands which secrete hormones into the bloodstream. Examples are the pituitary, pineal, adrenals and thyroid.

Epilepsy -- A disorder accompanied by periodic convulsions and loss of consciousness. It may be caused by many different conditions.

HCL -- Abbreviation for hydrochloric acid.

HHS - Abbreviation for Hiatal Hernia Syndrome.

Hiatal Hernia -- A protrusion of the stomach through a strain or torn diaphragm muscle.

Hiatal Hernia Syndrome -- The HHS is a syndrome that encompasses a multitude of symptoms dealing not only with digestive disturbances but numerous other problems. The major linking factor of these illnesses is the distribution of the vagus nerve and how it is affected by the interference of the stomach.

Hydrochloric Acid -- The only form of acid that is beneficial to the body. It is produced in the stomach by special cells and also produced by the vagus nerve. Without it, digestion of foods would be impossible.

Hypoglycemia -- (Low Blood Sugar) A condition of too little sugar in the blood that creates a multitude of Symptoms.

LBS -- Abbreviation for Low Blood Sugar (Hypoglycemia)

Lesion -- A change in tissue structures due to disease or injury. Many times tumors, ulcers and cuts are referred to as lesions.

Osteoarthritis -- Form of arthritis associated with cartilage and bone degeneration.

PMS -- Abbreviation for Pre-Menstrual Syndrome.

Pre-Menstrual Syndrome -- Condition in which symptoms could manifest such as fatigue, irritability, depression and inability to cope with life situations for one or two weeks occurring prior to the menstrual cycle.

Prostate -- Male gland behind outlet of the urinary bladder.

Temporo-Mandibular Joint -- This important joint is located just in front of the ears and is the junction of the lower jawbone and the temporal bone.

Thyroxin -- A hormone produced by the thyroid gland containing large quantities of iodine.

Thyroid Gland -- An endocrine gland located in the front of the neck which regulates body metabolism.

TMJ -- Abbreviation for Temporo-Mandibular Joint.

Triglycerides -- Fatty acid compound present in all people

Vagus Nerve -- The largest nerve in the body with many branches that begin in the brain and extend throughout most of the glands and organs. Nicknamed "the wanderer"

Vagotomy -- Surgically cutting the vagus nerve branch into the stomach to reduce excessive acidity.

INDEX

A

167

I

J

K

L

M

60, 61, 63, 65, 66, 68, 69, 70, 71, 74, 76, 77, 79, 81, 82, 85, 86, 88,
90, 91, 93, 94, 95, 96, 98, 101, 102, 103, 105, 106, 108, 109, 111,
112, 113, 114, 115, 116, 117, 118, 119, 125, 126, 127, 130, 131,
132, 134, 135, 136, 137, 138, 139, 140, 141, 142, 143, 144, 145,
146, 149, 151, 153, 154, 155, 156, 158, 159, 161, 165, 166
Stressi, 7, 12, 16, 32, 52, 57, 58, 73, 76, 77, 79, 80, 109, 135, 143, 144,
145, 162, 164

T

Temporo-Mandibular Joint .... i, 12, 16, 25, 90, 91, 166
Throat.................................... 11, 15, 22, 24, 95, 96, 117, 140
Thymus .... 71, 72, 73, 74, 75, 98, 162. *See Also* Gland(s), Thymus
Thyroid.. 28, 60, 66, 67, 87, 106, 165, 166. *See Also* Gland(s), Thyroid
Thyroxin.. 66, 166
TMJ .... *See* Temporo-Mandibular Joint
Triglyceride(s)................................. 30, 33, 34, 36, 60, 62, 63, 70, 166

U

Ulcer(s) .... i, 34, 42, 44, 45, 46, 116, 117, 153, 166
Urinary 12, 17, 25, 119, 166

V

Vagotomy... 33, 166
Vagus Nerve.... i, 5, 9, 10, 11, 15, 18, 20, 24, 28, 30, 31, 33, 34, 37, 38,
42, 44, 48, 52, 54, 55, 60, 70, 76, 93, 94, 95, 101, 103, 105, 140,
144, 154, 156, 162, 165, 166

W

Weight.. 38, 40, 60, 65, 66, 67, 137

BIOKINETIC FORMULAS
Created by Dr. Theodore Baroody to Promote Health
Through Alkaline-Forming Formulas
NUTRITIONAL SUPPLEMENTS

12-SYSTEMS SYNERGISTIC MULTIPLE
It is very difficult to find a multiple supplement that really creates balance within the body. I have tested over 100 different ones in the last 15 years. It has been my wish to formulate a truly balanced multiple food supplement for a long time. To do so, I used the 12 systems of Holographic Health as a model, because each substance fits into one of these categories. Each ingredient had to be balanced against the others in order to achieve a maximum overall synergistic health benefit in the body.

The 92 synergistically balanced ingredients in this formula are the result of many years of clinical experimentation. The 12 Systems Synergistic Multiple can be best described by the synergistic actions of each group, because each group is acting as a whole unit with its own purpose and thrust behind it.
Price: 100 Tablets - $19.95

ABSOLUTELY PURE L-GLUTAMINE
Glutamine is the most abundant free amino acid found in the muscles of the body. It is known as a brain food because it can readily pass the blood-brain barrier. It helps maintain the proper alkaline/acid balance in the body. It supplies the basic building blocks for DNA and RNA. It promotes mental ability and a healthy digestive tract. I use and recommend it for the following reasons:
1. It reduces shakiness and tremors (except in advanced Parkinson's disease).
2. It helps with depression, which I think is the result of excessive ammonia being generated in the body which is toxic to the brain. Glutamine can remove this.
3. For the instabilities of MS, ALS and their related cousin illness. I am not saying L-Glutamine will correct these conditions; I am only stating that it may help nutritionally. In fact, I have seen it do so many times.
4. It seems to have a great effect of epileptics, especially with petite minimal seizure. I have seen these minor seizures reduced to nothing with continuous glutamine usage.
5. It helps with all kinds of addictions, particularly addiction to alcohol.

Hiatal Hernia Syndrome

I use it as a powder because this increases its effectiveness and speed crossing the blood-brain barrier. The powder has very little taste. I recommend that you put it in your mouth and chase it down with water.

Price: 100 Powdered gram/3.5 Powdered oz - $19.95

ALKA-TRACE

(Liquid trace mineral drops for alkalizing fluids)

The body needs bioavailable trace minerals in order to operate. It needs some of these for practically every biochemical pathway. This is clear liquid preparation that is very low in sodium. I have used it successfully for over 15 years in practice. These life-giving droplets are very electrically conductive. Most importantly, they produce an alkaline reaction in fluids. You can put only 10 drops in water and get an 8.5 pH factor, which is very good. Therefore two purposes are served:

1) The body is given its much-needed trace elements.
2) The body is receiving an alkaline boost, which counteracts life-destroying waste acids in the body.

You can carry them in your pocket or purse and alkalize the water or other beverages that you drink daily.

1.25 ounces contain approximately 625 drops.

Price: 1.25 fl. oz. - $5.95

ALPHA-OMEGA

Essential fatty acids (EFAs) are the beginning and ending of all good nutritional programs. They are the fats that we cannot manufacture, but we need to live.

Symptoms of an EFA deficiency could include the following:

1. Growth retardation
2. Eczema
3. Hair loss
4. Liver degeneration
5. Heart problems
6. Behavioral problems
7. Kidney damage
8. Arthritis pains
9. Miscarriages
10. Excess sweating, with thirst
11. Sterility
12. Susceptible to infections
13. Weakness
14. Tingling sensations in arms and legs
15. Vision problems
16. Dry skin

In Alpha-Omega, we have good balance on most of the necessary EFA's. I use Alpha-Omega for all kinds of skin conditions coming from inside the body. If you have dry skin, eczema or any type of rash, you need EFA's. These are the most common symptoms I see of low EFAs.

Price: 100 Soft Gels - $26.95

AMISH HEALING WONDER OIL
(Secret Amish Formulation)

Every hundred years or so, a salve, balm, unction or formula of some sort comes along that just can't be topped. The Amish people are farming folk. One of the answers they found through generations of experimentation is the "Amish Healing Wonder Oil".

They use it on farm animals <u>and</u> for themselves. For the relief from open cuts (apply immediately), bruises, poison ivy and oak, any kind of bothersome skin patch, rare skin diseases, psoriasis, eczema, fungus under nails, and <u>especially</u> shingles.
Price: 4oz. Bottle - $7.95

ANEEM-AWAY

At the very least, during the change of each season (4 times a year), our bodies need reevaluation and a kick-start tonic that can transition us into the next cycle of months. The seasons are each related to one of the primary elements in our bodies, which are earth (winter), water (spring), fire (summer), and air (fall).

Edgar Cayce (considered the first modern voice of holistic medicine) recommended B's and iron together in his health research for people.

Studies have shown that iron significantly improves muscle function independent of positive blood tests for anemia. This tells me that many of us are walking around with subclinical B-complex/iron anemic syndromes.

There has been concern over the use of iron in the last few years; yet, survey upon survey consistently shows that iron deficiency is the <u>most common</u> nutritional deficiency, especially among children, women and older people.
Price: 8oz. Bottle - $9.95

ASPARA-CAN

The incredible health promoting properties of this vegetable so intrigued me that after doing research on it, I wrote the booklet, *Asparagus Can Do It for You.* As far as I can tell, everyone should be eating asparagus for a number of reasons. Two reasons are to improve heart balance and to prevent cancer. My book goes into detail on the many other things this tasty vegetable supplies. The extremely high alkaline-forming properties of asparagus are very beneficial to overall health. Aspara-Can was created because it is very difficult to get people to eat asparagus on a daily basis.
Price: 100 Capsules - $13.95

AT EEZ

This formula was made with one specific purpose: to rebalance and maintain a healthy overall nervous system. It will definitely help with sleep disorders (insomnia). Take as much as you need initially at bedtime to bring about good sleep.

AT-EEZ can be taken anytime, day or night if there is excessive nervousness, shaking, or hyperactivity. Give the nervous system plenty of time to heal. It does, but slowly. At first things may not seem to be better. They may even appear worse. Then things will start changing for the better. For mild conditions, try for 6 weeks without stopping to see if it will help. For severe conditions, try one year at least. If it is helping at all, don't stop. I know this seems a long time, but the nervous system requires it. In essence, it is like trying to repair your electrical house circuits while they are still on.

Price: 100 Tablets - $18.95

BABY-FLUSH

Some folks wanted to use Flush-Out with their children, but the children wouldn't put their faces in the water. Some adults also have the same problem, so I made up a stabilized solution of Flush-Out in distilled water. It comes in a one ounce clear plastic dropper bottle and can be used one of two ways; when held upright it will squirt up into the nose, when held upside down, it can be used as drops into the nose or eyes.

Price: 1.25oz. Bottle - $1.95

BACK-OFF

At least six times a month I find myself counseling afflicted clients about the dangers of the herpes virus and ways to deal with it. This disease is devastating physically, emotionally, and mentally. It hampers, intimidates, and many times destroys all sorts of personal relationships. It temporarily puts it in check. While hiding out at the level of the nervous system, it causes damages there. It can mutate. Evidence is emerging that several of the nerve related disorders, in any form, leaves a trail of minor to major destruction behind it. I have formulated something that I think may really help. I am not making claims of cure of treatment, however. Back-Off will not cure herpes.

Back off is designed to rebalance the body in its struggle with herpes infections. This includes simplex I (fever blisters and cold sores), and simplex II (genital herpes), shingles and other derivatives. It is not a substitute for medical treatment. The ingredients are things I have **see**n work over the years. Herpes is tough and aggressive. It takes a while to get it under control. Keeping it under control requires a lot of vigilance, particularly with genital herpes, but I feel it can be done.

Price 100 Tablets - $17.95

BEE POWERFUL

I have always considered bee products to be the most wholesome foods available to us. Both bee pollen and royal jelly have a complete pan-total complement of all the known B vitamins and their precursors in a perfectly balanced blend for the human body. Yet, I wanted more.

I sought to produce a product that contained not only bee pollen and royal jelly, but bee propulis as well. The source for this had to be local and fresh. Most royal jelly, propulis, and pollen products that you find are from overseas and have lost most, if not all, of their potency and freshness. I sought to know the beekeepers personally and that they themselves collected the product in its purest, freshest form. I also wanted something powerful enough to knock your socks off. I finally got the right combination. This is why I call it BEE POWERFUL.

It is a very precise combination of freeze-dried bee pollen, bee propulis, and bee royal jelly. I recommend this to anyone for their overall nutritional support.

Caution: A very tiny percent of the population are allergic to bee products, (about .5 of 1 percent). These poor souls are generally allergic to most everything. Many times, building up the use of bee products over a period of time can help all kinds of allergies. If you have doubts about this, start very slowly with the ingestion of this or any other bee products.

Price: 90 Capsules - $27.95

BEE THE BEST

Bee Pollen is the most complete and perfect whole super-food available to us as humans, reportedly containing over 185 nutritive substances.

Pollen is 35% protein. The bees put the collected grains of flower pollen into a single small pellet. Each pellet contains 2 million flower pollen grains and a teaspoonful contains 2.5 billion grains of flower pollen! Bee pollen contains every amino acid. It contains most every vitamin, but not limited to A, B1, B2, B3, B5, B6, B12, C, D, E, folic acid, rutin, inositol, and biotin, plus all the necessary minerals and trace minerals, calcium phosphorus, iron, copper, potassium, magnesium, manganese, silica, sulfur titanium, selenium, iodine, chlorine, boron, zinc and molybdenum. Also included are over 5,000 enzymes and co-enzymes. All of these substances are in a totally predigested, absorbable form.

Bee pollen's benefits are amazing. It helps skin, red blood cells, weight loss, allergies, sexual stamina, overall energy, PMS, enhances mental capacity, helps depression, hypertension, migraines, mental illness, eye fatigue, hair loss, activates the thymus gland, and some say increases longevity. I have been able to secure

Revised 1/2007

the finest high quality fresh bee pollen I have ever seen or tasted. This product is not dried or freeze dried. Be aware that if you live over 2 days from us by UPS, we will only ship Bee the Best by 2nd day freight.

Price: 4oz. Bottle - $7.95

B-WELL

B-Well is a B-complex liquid with all the same ingredients as Aneem-Away, but without iron. It also has a special B vitamin called DMAE (Dimenthylaminoethanol). DMAE is a brain stimulant for mood, intelligence, memory, depression, improves sleep and acts as an antioxidant.

If someone has only food allergies, they are helped more by the B-Well alone. If they have environmental allergies, they also have food allergies and this is helped by the Aneem-Away which contains both iron and B Vitamins with sodium ascorbate to "kick" the iron into the system very rapidly.

However, some folks are not iron deficient, yet have food allergies and the whole list of B vitamin deficiency symptoms. I am aiming B-Well toward all types that leave their victims leading very painful, disturbed lives of quiet desperation.

Price: 8oz. Bottle - $9.95

BLOOD HARMONIZER

This formula greatly assists with blood imbalances. I first made it to rebalance cholesterol and triglycerides, which it can do, but it is far more effective as a general blood circulation cleansing formula. I have seen it dissolve many blood clots and stagnations as they are referred to in Oriental medicine. Nosebleeds, blood impurities, certain kinds of headaches caused by old traumas where stagnation in the blood exists and bruises are all helped.

Also, as strange as it may sound, certain unseen health factors that can enter from the outside and are carried in the blood can be avoided or eliminated with the use of Blood Harmonizer. Particular forms of chemical and radioactive poisons so prevalent in our environment today will carry in the blood for years, sometimes before they deposit in the tissues, wreaking all manner of health imbalances that are barely detectable but dangerous, nevertheless. Blood Harmonizer rebalances these health imbalances if the poisons are caught before they deposit in the tissues.

Price: 100 Tablets - $19.95

CALCIUM PENETRATOR

Calcium is a requirement for all 60 trillion cells in the body. Yet, it is a difficult mineral to really understand. There are the many different theories of what kind to use and why. My chief concern has been true absorbability, especially in relationship to osteoporosis

Revised 1/2007

which is reaching epidemic proportions in people over 55. I am addressing almost every aspect of cellular interactions with Calcium Penetrator. Besides proper uptake into the bone, Calcium Penetrator could be helpful in tooth grinding, restless leg syndrome at night, and nighttime leg cramps. If you want to further improve your bone matrix, also add Pro-Tone and Cherry Gold. These will enhance the effectiveness of Calcium Penetrator even more.

Other calcium deficiency symptoms are: slow blood clotting, sluggish circulation, sensitive to moisture, afternoon headaches, dizzy in open air, staggering upon arising, palpitation under ascending stairs, varicose veins, icy sensation in spine, hemorrhages, soft bones, cysts, slimy salivation, sores that do not heal, lame ligaments, pus formation, discharges and insomnia.
Price: 100 Tablets - $16.95

CAMPHO-HEAL

Different forms of congestion are the primary cause of any and all pains and illnesses. Campho-Heal reaches deep into the body moving the more entrenched congestions that deal with stagnant energy, lymph and blood. It is for what the Chinese call "Yin" (Cold conditions). It is more "heating", but does not burn like capsicum and is very comforting. We use it for chronic, colder, deeper types of pain. It is especially good for chest congestions caused by colds.

Campho-Heal has such a penetrating ability that it works well to alleviate long-time aches and pains quickly. Use it on scars, particularly, as much energy is blocked at these sites.

The method of properly compounding these quantities of camphor is no longer commercially available and is not sold anywhere that I have seen. This old time "Yin" balancing formula we call Campho-Heal perfectly complements the Healing Wonder Oil, which is its "Yang" balancing counterpart.
Price: 2oz. Bottle - $6.95

CAN-CLEAR

The liver and colon are the main sites of excess poison accumulations that are the end result of our metabolism. Without proper eliminations there may still be waste poisons that persistently cling to the walls of the colon and want to "hang out" in the liver. Many of these are discarded cells are cancerous. Can-Clear regulates prostate, uterine and ovarian imbalances that might lead to more serious complications. It is, however, first and foremost a balanced bowel cleanser.
Price: 100 Tablets - $18.95

CHERRY GOLD

Arthritis and all related "-itis" conditions plague millions worldwide. It was my intent to combine certain natural elements that

Revised 1/2007

could greatly reduce the associated pain of arthritis while effectively supporting the possible rebuilding of bone, cartilage and ligaments. This has been achieved in Cherry Gold. Other interesting effects have been mild-to-marked relief from all kinds of pain -- headaches and muscle aches included. People report a mood-elevating factor as well. Some have dropped their anti-depressants.

I have used the knowledge of the enlightened 12th century lady, St. Hildegard of Bingen, as well as my own extensive research and experience in the making of this formula. I have seen results that are close to miraculous with it. If the arthritis is severe, and you are serious about getting well, I suggest NO intake of meat, white sugar, or alcohol for 90 days while taking Cherry Gold. Drink only distilled or high PH, alkaline-adjusted water for this period. Arthritis is a very acid condition. Eat lots of fruits and vegetables. These are alkaline-forming.

Price: 100 Capsules - $21.95

COLON-IZE

The human body is host to billions of micro-organisms. Some of these are good guys, and some are bad guys. There are more than 400 different species of bacteria in the gut, along with who knows the number of parasites and viruses.

One of the primary things I am addressing with Colon-ize is a serious issue called "Leaky Gut Syndrome". Even Edgar Cayce, considered the father of modern holistic medicine, spoke about the small intestines leaking poisons back into the general circulation of the body and being the primary cause of psoriasis.

When the large intestines (also called the colon) leaks through its walls, many other negative conditions can arise. Among these are chronic food and environmental allergies, lowered immune function, blood sugar disorders, a build up of cancer cell toxins, chemical sensitivities, irritable bowel syndrome, chronic arthritis, Crohn's disease, hepatitis, pancreatitis, and chronic fatigue.

I have always been attracted to colostrums. Thanks to a few individuals; it is finally getting the recognition it deserves as a health super-food. Colostrum contains an impressive list of immune factors and is involved in increasing bone and muscle mass, burning fat, healing of all body tissues and regulating the balance of fungus, bacteria, parasites and viruses in the body. It is further reported to relieve arthritis, reduce lupus levels, relieve allergies, asthma, help multiple sclerosis and herpes infections. However, I personally am making no claims for these conditions with Colon-ize. There is ample research to support what colostrum can do.

Also included in Colon-ize are five different types of lactobacillus. These help to stabilize and properly re-colonize the colon with "friendly bacteria" in just the right milligram amounts creating a "synergistic" blend with the colostrum.

I have purchased the highest possible grade of colostrums and acidophilus for Colon-ize.

Price: 100 Capsules - $21.95

COMPLETE-C

It is hard to find something for which vitamin C is not good. Studies show Vitamin C is effective in lowering the risks of developing cancers of the breast, cervix, colon, rectum, esophagus, larynx, lung, mouth, prostate, and stomach.

My purpose in making Complete-C is not just to provide another vitamin C supplement. There are a million of them out there now. The focus of this product is to be sure all areas of the C-complex are balanced. Most importantly, I want to repair, protect and sustain a very important metabolic system called the "Citric Acid Cycle" (Krebs cycle). This will lead to the beginning of all disease processes. Keeping this cycle operating at peak efficiency for as long as we can is a major priority.

Price: 100 Tablets - $17.95

DELETE

(For Relief from Outside Influences)

Holographic Health includes all facets of our health and life here. Just as I believe and have seen angels, so also do I believe and have seen the other spectrum of life. To help mitigate, protect and deal with some of these energies during this turbulent age of the prophecies, I have created "Delete". It is an anointing oil that is designed to give us protection and a little breathing room from these malevolent forces until whatever is going to happen, finally happens in this world.

Delete is composed of nine essential oils in almond base oil. These work in a synergistic manner for this imbalanced state.

Price: 1oz. Bottle - $14.95

DISINFECT

(For Ear Complaints)

If you or your children are having an earache or ear infection causing pain, and/or dizziness, you may want to try our all-natural-ingredient home remedy called *Disinfect*. Otitis media is the number one problem for children today, and more drugs are given for this than anything else. Most ear infections are the result of fungus.

Disinfect goes after these fungal infections with a vengeance; yet, it does so in a very safe, natural way that the body will accept. I have used this combination of oils for many years with success with my patients and family. I know it will work for you and your family, too. Shake it well and use 1 or 2 drops in each involved ear at night.

Revised 1/2007

Add a little piece of cotton in the ear to help hold the oil in, if necessary.
Price: 1/2oz. Bottle - $6.95

ENERGY UP

Energy Up nutritionally supports both men and women and targets the upper body hormones for the hypothalamus, thyroid, pituitary, and pineal. In women, it can also target the ovaries.
Price: 100 Tablets - $16.95

EYE-C

(For the Eyes)

The "Windows of the Soul" need not only to be cleaned on occasion, but also nourished and protected. Particularly, I was attempting to "feed the eye". One vitamin that the eye really loves is vitamin C. Not only does EYE-C help conjunctivitis (pink eye), tired, dry, red, and/or irritated eyes, but it also helps to heal styes. Headaches related to the eyes, both temple and frontal have also been eased by EYE-C. More serious eye disorders like cataracts, glaucoma, and macular degeneration have also been affected positively; however, no claims are made to help these conditions whatsoever.
Price: .5 fl. oz. - $6.95

FEEL-GOOD

Feel-Good nutritionally supports both men and women and basically targets the lower body hormones- the adrenal glands, cells of Leydig and testes in men, and the adrenal and cells of Leydig in women.
Price: 100 Tablets - $14.95

FLOW-THRU

The kidneys operate in a very rhythmic harmony with the heart. If this synchronization is disturbed, kidney-heart problems follow. Flow-Thru was created to rebalance this delicate balancing act between the kidneys and the heart.

The results vary. Though it may take a little longer, the excess water that is spilled from the kidneys into all the other tissues, causing swelling, organ interferences, and possible congestive heart disturbances, can be rebalanced. I often recommend Aspara-Can and or Kleen Sweep to be taken with Flow-Thru, if the heart is in a serious energetic imbalance.

Flow-Thru was also made to rebalance all manner of urinary, bladder and tract problems such as inflammation, gravel, and stones.
Price: 100 Tablets - $16.95

FLUSH OUT

Flush Out is an all-natural folk remedy used to relieve the mucous membranes and to help reduce the amount of infection, pollens, dust, chemicals and heavy metals that become trapped in the sinuses each day.

It is a facial bath that really works to help the sinuses. Patients rave about it! I recommend that you use it twice a day for best results.

Price: 2oz. Bottle - $7.95

FREE BREATH

After many clinical trials with the ingredients of this product, I am convinced that it will help to rebalance and rebuild the pulmonary system (lungs and bronchioles), and the sinuses. Many poisons and allergies are held deep in these sinus cavities and cause continuous mucous and drainage. It appears to reduce the desire to smoke, according to how many you take. Clinically, I have seen migraines helped by Free Breath. To assist with trapped particles in the sinuses, I recommend the sinus facial bath called Flush Out that will help to further reduce these allergens, as well as sinusitis. I highly suggest that you use both of these products together.

Price: 100 Tablets - $17.95

FRESH START

It was brought to my attention that we had the need for a good totally natural safe feminine hygiene product. I began to question the ladies about this and sure enough, they told me how great the need really was.

I began testing different ideas and came up with a wonderful feminine hygiene formula. It does not seem to be drying and yet, if used enough, will rebalance the problems that occur.

I find Fresh Start helpful for many types of problems. These include acute to chronic infections, burning, itching, vaginal scarring and lower pelvic pain. It can be used much more frequently than other hygiene products and seems to balance the pH.

We find that maintenance usage not only reduces current problems but also seems to help with prevention of other situations. It is a complicated formulation; yet from what I see on the drug store shelves it is quite reasonably priced.

I have also used it in place of Flush Out for sinus problems. It works great for that, too. Put it directly in the nostrils without dilution for the best results.

Price: 2oz. Bottle - $11.95

FUNGAL FOE

Authorities state that 80 million (1 out of 3) Americans may have too much candida albicans in their systems. Candida is a fungal yeast infection. The lists of problems that candida overgrowth may cause are shocking. The tricky thing about candida is that it is a naturally occurring yeast in our bodies.

It responds to the many toxins causing bacterial, viral and parasitic mass production. Even if the immune system is strong enough to handle the multiple critters birthed by the candida toxins, the candida infection itself still stays intact systematically in the body, creating havoc on all levels. Then, the entrenched candida simply begins again. More and more toxins are produced while the overworked immune system struggles to readjust and salvage what it can from onslaught to onslaught. Meanwhile, you, the candida victim, just get sicker and sicker from one infection to another until a total collapse becomes imminent.

Price: 100 Tablets - $19.95

GREAT GUMS

Infections that get around the teeth roots are treacherous and sometimes difficult to eradicate. Many times, just using Great Gums several times a day helps some of the tough infections, gingivitis, and pyorrhea (Riggs disease) problems.

Price: 2oz. Bottle - $10.95

HEART-LINE

Hypertension, or high blood pressure, is a dangerous problem facing a huge segment of both the male and female population, approximately 60 million Americans. It not only afflicts the middle to older age citizens, but is now beginning its insidious creep down into younger and younger ages.

Lately, I have been made aware of what my teachers call "subtle heart attacks that occur in women". It appears that the heart conditions in women go undiagnosed or dismissed more often than I realized. Ladies, if there is a deep ache and deep pinching pressure between the breasts and yet nothing shows with medical testing, I suspect a real problem is in the making. Differential diagnosis that I find is to rule out Hiatal Hernia Syndrome. If this is not it, why not take about 6 to 8 Heart-Line and see if the pain subsides? If it does, be suspicious.

Price: 100 Tablets - $18.95

HEMORR-MEND

Hemorrhoids bother a great deal of the population. There are different types. Some bleed, some protrude, some are internal, some hurt and some don't. All are problematical.

Revised 1/2007

It appears that what causes their presence is a rather complicated matter. It is not just excessive lifting or constipation. It is involved with many interrelated body systems. For example, coccyx problems and bowel infections, energetic imbalances, and strangely enough even some ear infections are also sometimes involved.

Hemorr-Mend is made to help all of these. It takes time to heal these problems. Watch your progress, as you use it daily; it is completely safe for all ages.

Price: 1.25 oz. - $4.95

H.H.S. FORMULA
(Hiatal Hernia Syndrome)

This interactive formulation is the result of working with thousands of clinical cases of Hiatal Hernia Syndrome involvement. Since publication of my book, Hiatal Hernia Syndrome: The Mother of All Illness, every kind of digestive disorder has been referred to me.

When I was creating this food supplement, all of this information plus every gland, organ and valve relating to the improvement and perfection of all digestive functions were considered. After careful experimentation, my clients, family, and friends are now benefiting. I have received hundreds of reports from people nationwide who have gained relief from this product.

Price: 100 Capsules - $14.95

H.H.S. STOMACH EGG

After 20 years of giving people instructions on how to work on their Hiatal Hernia Syndrome for themselves, I think I have found a better answer. Some people report that it is just too painful on their hands to do the HHS maneuver as I describe it in my book, because of hand problems. I discovered that this particular size wooden egg fits perfectly under the rib cage for pulling down and correcting the HHS. Instructions included.

Price: Each Egg - $9.95

HOLOPATHICS

According to physics, all matter is made up of energy. The body is a group of energy signatures working in energetic union with each other. When they are balanced, we feel good. When they are not, we feel bad. Every state of health has a frequency. What we have done is to create frequencies that will bring certain conditions back into balance. This does include everything.

We use an electronic device that generates completely harmless energy signatures and puts them into milk sugar pills. These little wonder pills have no side effects. They either work or not. No promises are made.

Hiatal Hernia Syndrome

To use the drops, pour a few into the lid and then place under tongue. Do not touch them with your hands. They come in ½ oz. bottles of approximately 150 pills each. We can also put these in water, if you prefer.

Ask us for a copy of the complete catalog for a list of the holopathics, or you can find them online.

Price: ½ oz. Bottle - $5.95

INFECT AWAY

When we let ourselves get out of balance, all manner of infective processes, allergies, bacteria, fungus, parasites and viruses constantly try to help us return to a balanced state. When any of these "bugs" or critters overproliferate they can cause great distress to us. If we are not on a nutritional program of regeneration, they will further weaken the immune system.

Infect Away was formulated to support the immune system in dealing with any and all infections. Think of it as a natural antibiotic, anti-fungal, anti-parasitic and anti-viral therapeutic food supplement. To complete the balance in this formula, all four elements within the immune system: earth, water, fire, and air are addressed in correct ratio to each other. The results speak for themselves, as letters flood in testifying how the formula has worked on all types of infection.

Price: 100 Capsules - $16.95

IN-SYNC

Pain is a symptom of other, most of the time, deeper problems. To just reduce or eliminate the pain symptoms without also taking into consideration the effect this will have on the body's many systems is short sighted.

What I have attempted to do with In-Sync is to create a balance within the 12 systems that will bring a temporary lessening or elimination of different kinds of pain. Therefore, this is not a painkiller in the traditional sense of the word, but more a pain-leveler or pain synchronizer throughout the 12 systems of the body. It provides mediation between what is causing the pain and the pain itself, while allowing the organ of involvement to re-synchronize certain aspects of its abnormal function.

Price: 100 Tablets - $18.95

KLEEN SWEEP

The number one health problem worldwide is heart and circulatory involvements. We are constantly faced with the dilemma of how to keep our precious vessels clear and elastic, and our hearts as healthy as possible from all viewpoints.

Involved in many heart and circulatory disorders are heavy metals, man-made chemicals, radiation and occasionally, geopathologically-caused toxic residues that have lodged any and everywhere throughout the body. Kleen Sweep was formulated to address all these nutritional needs, while simultaneously re-oxygenating the entire body through the 4 elements, Earth, Water, Fire, and Air.

Price: 100 Capsules - $17.95

MAGNESIUM PENETRATOR

Magnesium Penetrator was made to keep the soft tissues in proper balance--that is, supple, young, and free from excess waste products that cause pain and rapid aging. Because of our acid-forming life styles including diet, lack of exercise, and unbelievable amount of stressors, our much-needed calcium migrates from the hard tissues (bones) to the soft tissues. This causes premature aging in the arteries, calcification results in hardening of the arteries. In the heart, it results in heart problems, in the joints, calcification causes arthritis. In the kidneys, it causes kidney stones. In the eyes, calcification causes cataracts. In the hair, it causes brittleness, and in the brain, senility. In the cells, calcification causes a blockage of protein synthesis.

So many clients have asked me why I did not have a calcium-magnesium combination formula. The answer is simple. Calcium and magnesium compete for absorption sites in the small intestines. They are antagonistic to each other, so if you take them at the same time, at least some of what you expect to get out of the supplement will be lost. If you are going to take both Calcium Penetrator and Magnesium Penetrator, then take the Magnesium Penetrator in the morning and Calcium Penetrator in the evening. I made Calcium Penetrator to reach the bones, not to stop and pile up in the soft tissue. Both of these products are vital to the human body, particularly if they are taken at the right times.

Price: 100 Tablets - $17.95

MAGNETS

Magnets have been used for healing since ancient times. Back then, they were called "lodestones" and considered magical. Today, magnets are still magical in their ability to help with physical pain. These are inexpensive, powerful, round magnets. They are marked by an indentation in the center of one side so you can tell north pole from the south pole. Magnetism penetrates everything. Just tape them on a painful spot and see if it helps.

PUT THE SMOOTH SIDE AGAINST THE SKIN.

Price: Per Each Approximately 4000 gauss - $1.95

MINOTAUR

The Minotaur is an ancient Greek, half-human, half bull with incredible strength. It represents the power within us to constantly improve ourselves through greater inner strength and musculoskeletal focus.

Minotaur works for both men and women. It supports every kind of situation in which a person wishes to improve his muscle, joint and connective tissue, strengthen and tone. This applies to both athletes and non-athletes. It definitely helps muscular and skeletal imbalances anywhere in the body to begin to stabilize and finally hold.

Clinically, everyone using Minotaur, from spring gardeners to weight lifters, people working in construction, doing aerobics, or those just trying to get in shape have received great benefit. Musculoskeletal pains have been greatly reduced, or in many cases disappeared. My workout partner, a world-class lifter, had a terrible rotator cuff injury with a spur. He suffered steady, intractable pain for a year. After two days on Minotaur, the pain disappeared. After several weeks he is lifting better than ever. He reports that his arms and chest feel stronger and more pumped, even when not working out.

I can assure you that this product is absolutely pure. The chemical assay reports confirm this and are available with this product. The ingredients are free from any kind of binders or fillers. They work much better together as a powder, which is why I've made it available to you in this form. Take it in water or juice (except orange and grapefruit), or as I recommend by just putting the powder directly into your mouth and chase it down with water. It has little or no aftertaste, if swallowed quickly.

Price: 100 Grams - $12.95 / 250 Grams - $25.95
500 Grams - $46.95 / 1000 Grams - $79.95

MOOD MENDER

After doing research I was stunned to find out that 11 million plus Americans are newly reported to have "depression" each year. The number of prescriptions written for mood enhancers and depression lifters is even far greater for the same period of time. A huge number of people are on these substances. A recent survey indicated that nearly ½ of the US population had undergone a serious, diagnosable, psychiatric condition.

Mood Mender is aimed at re-balancing the brain nutritionally and to stabilize it by a totally natural method.

Price: 100 Tablets - $19.95

MYO-MAJESTIC

Revised 1/2007

MYO-MAJESTIC is a muscle sculpting food supplement which contains MYO-MY! and MINOTAUR mixed together. It has all the same benefits as these two separately but will not bulk you up as quickly as just the MINOTAUR will.

I compounded it in response to certain male and female needs that could tolerate lower doses of MINOTAUR but were not able to see the results they wanted as quickly. As I have stated before, some women cannot take MINOTAUR because of water retention. MYO-MAJESTIC does not seem to cause this water retention in women, yet gives them the energy and strength.

There is also a group of men who are taking ACE inhibitors for their heart. These drugs hold onto creatine in the body, so they cannot take too much creatine. MYO-MAJESTIC is the answer for this, too. They get a small amount of creatine but not enough to cause any real overuse problems. The body repairing properties of MYO-MAJESTIC are noteworthy.

Price: 100 grams - $16.95

MYO-MY!

MYO-MY! is a muscle-sculpting food supplement. (MYO means muscle and MY! is the response you can get when others see you.) It will build muscle also, but I use it as a repairing and sculpting food.

It seems to reduce cortisol, which causes mid-section belly weight. Even though it is used to help bodybuilders recover much more quickly and build more lean muscle while reducing fat produced by cortisol, people who do not lift weights can benefit equally.

The reason is this. The body is in a constant state of muscle breakdown. This is called catabolism. If the body is not fed properly, it will seek branched chain amino acids (BCAAs), which are found in already existing muscle and cannibalize them for its survival. Thus, you have muscle wasting, which is very common after the age of forty in everyone. In order to stop this insidious march of an ever-weakening musculature, you need to supply the body with the proper balance of BCAAs.

BCAA supplementation has been reported to decrease exercise-induced protein degradation and/or muscle enzyme release (an indicator of muscle damage), possibly by promoting an anti-catabolic hormonal profile. The availability of BCAAs during exercise has been theorized to help with fatigue. During endurance exercise, BCAAs are taken up by the muscles rather than the liver in order to contribute to oxidative metabolism.

MYO-MY! works for both men and women. It supports every kind of situation in which a person wishes to improve their muscle tone. This applies to both athletes and non-athletes. It definitely

helps muscular and skeletal imbalances anywhere in the body to begin to stabilize and finally hold.
Price: 100 grams - $18.95

NAIL-WELL

Nail fungus is made up of tiny organisms (tinea unguium, onychomycosis) that can infect fingernails and toenails. The nails of our fingers and toes are very effective barriers. This barrier makes it quite difficult for a superficial infection to invade the nail.

Once an infection has set up residence, however, the same barrier that was so effective in protecting us against infection now works against us, making it difficult to treat the infection. More than 35 million people in the United States get this fungus. The fungus lives underneath the nail. The nail provides a safe place for the fungus and protects it while it grows, since fungus like dark and damp places. This is why it's hard to reach and stop nail fungus.

The treatment of nail fungus is slow but if you are consistent, Nail-Well will kill the fungus without it coming back. It is a realistic expectation to get a reasonable improvement in a six month to one year span.
Price: .5 oz - $11.95

OUCH-AWAY!

Ouch-Away! is a spray-on blend of nine different natural oils for immediate pain relief. Just as Campho-Heal and Healing Wonder Oil deal with the different forms of congestion, Ouch-Away removes superficial circulatory imbalances that cause pain. While congestive problems directly affect the lymphatics more and are deeper imbalances, the circulatory system can hold blockages in it that are closer to the surface. It is these that Ouch-away targets efficiently and effectively. It works so well that in many cases the pain relief is felt on the spot. It will surprise you how fast it works. Not all aches and pains can be alleviated rapidly if they have been there for a while. If you notice any relief whatsoever, then in time the relief will be very significant. Use as much as needed. There do not seem to be any side effects.

I would use Ouch-Away in conjunction with one or both of the Yin-Yang decongestive formulas (Healing Wonder Oil and/or Campho-Heal) if pain persists. I was amazed when I saw how fast it worked on even the most stubborn pains.

This formula is complex to blend and is a mixture of five completely natural carrier oils and four essential oils. There are a number of energy signatures in it that accentuates its effectiveness, in my opinion. I would be interested to hear your comments on how this does for you. I carry a bottle with me about all the time, because somebody always needs it.   *Price: (Oil) 2 oz./SPRAY Bottle $14.95*

PAN-GEST

Pan-Gest was formulated to assist in every part of the digestive cycle. It is for problems with bloating, indigestion, gall bladder, pancreas, and liver pain, in particular. Anything that has to do with the pancreas will be addressed with Pan-Gest, including all types of blood sugar imbalances. Pan-Gest is designed to nutritionally support deeper digestive problems and the many offshoots that it might cause.

HHS Formula is a wonderful adjunct to take with Pan-Gest, if you have these deeper problems. Pan-Gest does not address the Hiatal Hernia Syndrome or upper stomach problems the way the HHS Formula does, nor is it particularly helpful with upper stomach ulcers. Use HHS Formula for these.

Think of Pan-Gest as the heavy artillery division of digestive support. It is also helpful for inflammations anywhere in the body.

Price: 100 Tablets: $21.95

PARA-GO-WAY

No one is exempt. We all have parasites. The irony of this is that just like all the other critters such as bacteria, fungus and viruses, we need them. It is a necessity that parasites remain in balance with the rest of our system; otherwise, they overpopulate and pave the way for other outside destructive parasites to enter. This is what is happening today because of the toxic state of the world, our poor diets, and impacted colons. This creates a great breeding ground for all sorts of "nasties".

Very few formulas seemed to check out as well for the body. I finally figured out the reason: 1) the pills were too big; 2) our old standbys like black walnut have become not as effective as they used to be; 3) I wanted to ensure that while I was balancing out the parasite population that the other eleven systems stayed in balance also.

Price: 240 Tablets - $17.95

PINK LADY

(A Trans-Dermal Crème for Vitamin B₁₂ Imbalances)

If I had to pick any single vitamin that is most needed by the body and most deficient in the entire world population, it would unquestionably be B_{12}. The need I see for B_{12} in my clientele alone over the past 20 years has been alarming.

B_{12} is usefully absorbed only by 1% from taking supplements or sublingually (under the tongue), no matter what you hear. The clinical symptoms don't disappear. It is best absorbed by liquid injections. These definitely work because they bypass all aspects of the digestive system, go directly into the blood and to proper places in the body in just moments. Unfortunately, B_{12} injections are by prescription only and 99.5% of our medical authorities don't believe mild to moderate B_{12} deficiencies are a problem or they simply refuse to write the prescription. So, I made a B_{12} crème.

It is simple to use and very pink, thus the name "Pink Lady". Using a carrier system, I was able to get the B_{12} effectively through the skin and into the blood completely bypassing the digestive process in a matter of seconds. This is a nontoxic, hypo-allergenic crème.

Give it at least 60 days to see, though it seems to work quickly. Just rub it on anywhere, except the face. It sure beats taking injections, if you can get them at all, or taking B_{12} food supplements that everybody in the trade knows don't work.

According to medical texts the need for B_{12} increases during periods of high stress and pregnancy. Another interesting fact about B_{12} is that it is the only vitamin that also contains essential mineral elements. There is some research that B_{12} is important for the prevention and treatment of autoimmune imbalances as well. This is where the immune system goes haywire and produces antibodies that fight against the body's own tissues.

Price: 1.25 oz. Crème - $9.95

POTASSIUM PENETRATOR

Potassium is an extremely vital mineral; yet, it is given very little attention in health circles. This is baffling when we examine all the symptoms that a low potassium level causes.

We use so much sodium in the form of salt in our food that potassium imbalances have reached epidemic proportions. The primary example of this is hypertension (high blood pressure). So many more people have hypertension worldwide now than 50 years ago that it is appalling.

Chemically, we know that an increase in sodium will elevate blood pressure. In Potassium Penetrator, I have formulated the six (6) different types of the most absorbable forms.

Potassium Penetrator can be used along with your heart program of Heart-Line, Kleen Sweep, and Magnesium Penetrator.

Potassium assists so many different imbalances that it is alarming. Chronic Fatigue responds well to potassium, as well as all sorts of brain disorders.

My principle reason for liking potassium so much is because it is an excellent alkalizer. It is my experience in clinical situations that the more accumulated acid in your system, the sicker you become.

Price: 100 Tablets - $17.95

PROTECTOR

Protector was created to help us men prevent these oncoming possibilities, as well as increase our natural sex drive and libido. It will definitely assist in the rebalancing of BPH.

Prostate problems (BPH) and loss of sexual expression can go hand in hand. We definitely want to maintain both aspects of our health as long as possible.

Price: 100 Tablets - $19.95

PRO-TONE

Natural Progesterone is a most interesting hormone. Not only does it stabilize numerous conditions in females, but it also is supportive to males. Neither sex can live well without it.

It is from a plant sterol that is converted to the identical substance. It restores sexual energy, balances cell oxygen levels, raises body temperature by improving thyroid function, a natural diuretic and anti-depressant, aids in protection against fibrocystic breasts, uses fat for energy, is necessary for embryo and fetus survival, and is a precursor of other sex hormones such as estrogen and testosterone. It relieves vaginal dryness and helps prevent cardiovascular vasospasms. When used by itself or with Women's Booster, I have seen it dramatically help pre-menstrual syndrome.

Price: ¾ oz. jar - $11.95

RACKET-FREE

There are times in the lives of certain individuals when they simply must face an undisputable truth-- THEY SNORE!
I have seen bruised and battered men walk into my office more than once because their partners had pummeled them in the back and legs with forceful blows of the fist and merciless toes into the calves.

I thought at first that this was a way their partners were just getting even with them for who knows what, until it happened to me. Though my ex-wife was gentle, her pinches and punches were definitely not love taps.

Relationship problems abound from snoring. Spouses move to separate bedrooms. The amount of sleep hours lost, work hours poorly performed, and accidents of all types occurring because of snoring partners will never be known. I am sure the price is in the billions of lost dollars.

Then, there is the dark side of snoring. The condition known as sleep apnea can ruin a person's health. Snoring has not been medically linked by research to sleep apnea, but it is blatantly apparent to doctors dealing with this problem that more often that not, snoring is one of the primary symptoms.

Racket-Free is an oral-spray for snoring. Like everything else in this product guide, it was made for my patients because of their

Revised 1/2007

needs. It is not a 100% snore stopper. In severe cases, with or without a diagnosis of sleep apnea, Racket-Free lowers the volume by a full 75%. In moderate cases, it moves to 85-90%. In mild cases, it is usually 100% successful. Of course, there are always those that it will not help at all.

Racket-Free has to be used nightly. There is evidence that it has a cumulative effect. Perhaps there is some actual healing of the problem.

Price: 2 oz. Spray Bottle - $19.95

SENSES

Senses has been formulated to deal with infections that hamper primarily the ears. Ear infections are so common among children that they may be thought of as a type of ongoing epidemic. Antibiotics, dispensed like candy to children, are becoming less and less effective.

Ear infections in the adult population are almost as common as they are in children; however, many of these adult ear infections go unrecognized. This is because they can manifest in usual ways not easily identifiable as coming from the ear. Many are related to headaches, TMJ problems, neck pain and a group of different kinds of shoulder pains. These symptoms can display themselves even with no particular pains in the ear being evident, so the practitioner often misses ear infections as a source of these discomforts and treats other areas instead.

Senses also has a positive effect on the eyes and nasal passages. The eyes are often the victim of ear infections that migrate over into them. Senses addresses these deeper stubborn head infections that seem to linger on and on causing the ears, eyes, smell and taste to be compromised.

Price: 100 Tablets - $17.95

SUNGOLD

Sungold is hypoallergenic crème containing a high amount of Folic Acid, B_{12}, and B_6. Each dab, the size of a thumbnail, provides an easily obtainable form of these vitamins. They can be utilized by the body by rubbing them onto the feet or abdomen.

I formulated Sungold for several reasons:
1. I believe we are in a B_{12} crisis, and folic acid helps to hold B_{12} in the body as well as working as a synergistic to B_{12}.
2. I find that folic acid has been greatly underestimated in its need. If it is needed for a developing baby, what about afterwards? We are still growing until age 20. After that, the body needs a large amount of folic acid to maintain all the changes that we go through.

3. Most all of the B-vitamins are eaten up in our bodies from the extraordinary amount of stress that we all suffer from today.
4. There is quite a body of research that talks about the amino acid homocysteine, not cholesterol, as being the major reason for heart disease. Homocysteine causes severe atherosclerosis. This was discovered by Dr. Kilmer McCully in 1969. Further, he found a most interesting discovery. All patients with high homocysteine levels were also low in three specific B vitamins. These are folic acid, B12 and B6.
5. I find that this combination works great against all types of infections. It is excellent for those who do not like to swallow pills. This is also preferable for children.

Price: 1.25 oz. - $11.95

SYMMETRY

Antioxidants are the guardians of our bodies. This formula is designed for the tougher, deeper imbalances that strike the body through our immune/nervous/circulatory system connections. It is also for preventative maintenance to help stabilize all of our systems against the ravages of time.

Although we all will age, this formula aims to mitigate many of the factors associated with oxidation and make the aging process easier by influencing longevity at the cellular level. It is also for the degenerative nerve conditions like multiple sclerosis, Parkinson, and ALS.

The circulatory ability must be improved to carry the necessary immune factors to the needed areas. Without proper nerve functions, nothing operates properly. These systems must be kept at peak performance as long as possible. These three together form a protective triangle for the body to operate within. They also support the subtle nervous system affecting the areas called the Ida, Pingala, and Sushuma. It brings these into balance joining the energy centers of the coccyx to the ones in the cranium. No claims of diagnosis or medical treatment are made. This is simply a nutritional support for the body.

The immune system is under such attack today. Symmetry is designed as an extremely potent antioxidant formula to relieve the stressors placed onto it. Another feature is its ability to support the vessels surrounding the heart. This may help with general support for the entire nervous system as well. It may bring relief from the tensions of the day through nervous system support and restructuring.

Price: 100 Tablets - $19.95

THE RECIPE
(Natural Cough Syrup)

Revised 1/2007

Hiatal Hernia Syndrome

Mr. Brett, a senior citizen from rural Georgia, introduced me to a cough syrup recipe that works on even the toughest cases. He claims it is an old concoction made of all natural ingredients. I can say that I personally use it, and my little girl loves it so much she tries to drink the whole bottle!

Shake it up well; then take a little at a time in the mouth and hold it there. It will naturally seep down the throat and work wonders.

Price: 4oz. Bottle - $7.95

TRI-FORCE

Tri-Force is made to coordinate and support this triad:
1. Power
2. Courage
3. Wisdom

Deficiency symptoms of these areas are the same as the thyroid symptoms under Energy Up because the pituitary controls the thyroid. Sometimes the client does not have a low thyroid, they have a pituitary affecting the thyroid.

Pituitary weaknesses are and can include:

1) Excessive urination
2) Left side head pain(left cervical)
3) Chronic headaches at the level of the eyes
4) Overweight
5) Non-insulin responsive diabetic
6) Sexual problems
7) Weakening of ligaments, bones and tenderness
8) Mental illness in self or family
9) Inability to be coordinated at night
10) Mental fatigue
11) Low energy
12) Cold hands and feet
13) Loss of head hair
14) Numbness and tingling sensations
15) A feeling of weak upper body strength and
16) Brittle nails.

Price: 100 Tablets - $17.95

WEIGHT LOSS - A BALANCED APPROACH

Weight problems are complex. They cover every aspect of the psychological as well as physiological makeup of a person; therefore, I have created an approach that addresses this problem from a multitude of directions. I have been asked about dietary approaches to weight imbalances since my first day as a doctor. After 20 years of watching patients and friends suffer from the mental, emotional and physical pain that excessive weight causes in all areas of their lives, I feel I have a safe answer. Trim-Silver is for nighttime weight reduction. This supplement is made to relax the body, burn fat during the night, and simultaneously curb the appetite.

Also included are recommendations for exercise, low carbohydrate eating, food combining, alkaline/acid forming ratios and drinking water.

It is important for anyone wishing to use Trim-Silver to understand that I am not holding myself out as a weight-loss guru, nor do I stand alone in my ideas. Through careful observation over the last 20 years, I have determined which weight-loss approaches seemed to work while keeping the body in balance, and why. I have combined the ideas from which I feel you can benefit. I have then added my own knowledge and experience to the process.

This is why I am recommending that you use two other products to insure that you will stay in balance during the time you are losing weight. Both of these have proven to us clinically that they will assist in weight loss on their own, but I do not sell them just for this purpose. These two products are 12 Systems Synergistic Multiple and Extreme Greens. These will provide the missing needs in your diet when you change it, without adding anything into the diet that will increase weight.

A fourth supplement, Can-Clear, may be needed if you have trouble with constipation. If you are not going often enough, acid waste poisons accumulate quickly causing all manner of illnesses and weight problems. Excess weight is held in the body by these poisons and other tissue acid wastes. They hold water and fat in the cells and in-between the cells. To enhance weight loss metabolism, we want to reduce these poison by-products from the body.

Price: Balanced Weight Loss System: All Three Bottles - $54.95

WIPE-OUT

Wipe-Out is for seriously resistant infective imbalances that are not responding to other approaches, such as Infect-Away, Fungal Foe, Para-Go-Way, Free Breath and Senses. We are seeing the re-emergence of many older diseases. It appears that our over-utilization of synthetic drugs has created a whole new set of stronger than ever monsters. Many strains are mutating into more and more powerful forms. We have had excellent results with many of these difficult imbalances with this product.

Wipe-Out is a powder that combines many factors nutritionally and energetically. It tastes about like a sweet tart. Do not mix it with citrus juices. You might get a healing crisis (Herxheimer reaction) from this product. I can guarantee that all of the ingredients are natural and are the highest quality available.
Price: 100 grams - $19.95

WOMEN'S BOOSTER

This formula is specifically for women. It contains a balanced set of ingredients to support mostly the ovaries and uterus, but can also strengthen practically the entire hormonal system.   In our modern times when artificial hormones are causing cancer, this safe, natural formula has been shown to help with female imbalances.
Price: 100 Tablets - $17.95

ZINC PENETRATOR

Zinc has a large variety of functions in which it participates. It is related to the normal absorption and action of vitamins, especially the B complex. It is involved in at least 25 known enzymes associated with metabolism. Zinc is a prime component of insulin, and it is needed to break down alcohol.

In fact, zinc has so many applications in clinical nutrition that it is difficult to pick just one area in which to focus this supplement. I have chosen to direct the formulation of this supplement toward skin imbalances. Dr. Jonathan Wright has had great success with atopic eczema, also called atopic dermatitis, and eczematous dermatitis when using zinc. The primary symptom of this kind of eczema is that it appears on the skin in front of the elbows and behind the knees. I use zinc for any skin problem I find.

Other zinc deficiencies include:

ulcers	diabetes	Hodgkins disease
prostatitis	infertility	arteriosclerosis
cystic fibrosis	alcoholism	slow wound healing
hypoglycemia	cirrhosis	night blindness
low libido	low energy	depression
canker sores	baldness	brittle nails and hair
dandruff	sore knees	reduced taste and smell
sore hip joints	stretch marks	white spots on fingernails

Price: 100 Tablets - $18.95

BOOKS AND MEDIA

ASCENSION: BEGINNER'S MANUAL

LOVE. Love is the total, the beginning and ending of this process called ASCENSION -- our evolutionary destiny. This means to change every molecule of the physical body to light and thereby immortalize it. This book is a complete "how-to" treatise based on the author's years of out-of-body and lucid dream experiences since childhood, combined with his own clinical research showing the link to health. It is divided into the five stages of growth with diet, cleansing, exercise, and contemplation.

223 pages, ISBN: 0-9619595-1-7 Price: $12.95

"They have been distributed all across the country – coast to coast, border to border and then some....Canada and even Nigeria with the wife of a chief there!" Unity Village, Mo

ASCENSION: BEGINNER'S MANUAL II

We are never anywhere except the beginning. ASCENSION: Beginner's Manual II is dedicated to demonstrating this fact. It is written from the viewpoint of quantum mechanics, biomagnetics, and their relationships to the One Great Law of LOVE. According to our present understanding of science, we are giant interlocking vibratory energy patterns -- a vast network of personal information that forms us as living, conscious entities.

This volume explores many avenues in which to consider the ASCENSION process. It unites and expands the knowledge of the first manual, providing both a historical background and a current methodology that is both accessible and applicable to our present time.

205 pages, ISBN: 0-9619595-9-2 Price: $17.95

ASPARAGUS CAN DO IT FOR YOU

Dr. Baroody has been very excited to confirm many earlier reports regarding the health benefits of asparagus, known to be beneficial as an immune system builder and for heart arrhythmia conditions. This booklet includes well documented client reports and easy to follow directions on how to prepare and take asparagus in either fresh or capsule form.

52 pages, ISBN: 0-9619595-4-1   Price: $4.95

THE BROTHERHOOD OF INTUITION

This small booklet is to guide you in the development of your intuition. I started to discontinue this booklet but have received so many requests for it recently that I decided to include it in the catalog.

27 Pages, ISBN: 0-9619595-0-9   Price: $3.95

80%/20% ALKALINE-ACID CHART

A wonderful doctor in New Zealand appreciated my book, Alkalize or Die, so much that she created this colorful, artistic, and easy-to-read poster for learning correct food balancing for superior health. There is a wealth of useful information on the back as well! This chart is appropriate for framing or just tacking to the refrigerator. Many people are using them as place mats!

Full-color, heavy, gloss-coated and laminated   Price: $14.95

HOLOGRAPHIC HEALTH -- VOLUME I
Earth Element, Holotherapy

Holographic Health is a complete paradigm of wellness. It is a multifaceted, multi-disciplinary approach to superior health. The basic premise is that at the center of our being, we are immortal souls. As souls, we manifest physically and energetically through four elemental pathways. These are, air, fire, water and earth, respectively.

The Soul attracts to itself these four elements, thereby creating a living being. Each of these elements manifests as a different part of our complete makeup. The air element delivers our intuition. Fire ushers forth the mind. Water yields our emotions. Earth gives us a physical body.

This is the first of four volumes. It encompasses the earth element and gives the practitioner and layperson alike a solid foundation upon which to help others who are suffering with structural and connective tissue problems. Through these pages and in coordination with the other volumes, students of Holographic Health will gain a comprehensive knowledge of our holistic nature.

Recommended for Licensed Professionals:
327 Pages, ISBN: 0-9619595-5-X
650 Photos   Explanatory diagrams and charts.   Price: $39.95

HOLOGRAPHIC HEALTH -- VOLUME II
Fire Element, Holosomatics

Volume II is a series of four books by Dr. Baroody which outline the testing methods, procedure, and protocol for his Holographic Health Testing Program. It is illustrated with hundreds of pictures, diagrams, charts, and easy-to-follow directions on how to muscle test, check the body for primary imbalances, and how to balance them, if weakened.

Recommended for Licensed Professionals:
535 pages, ISBN: 0-9619595-8-6
450 Photos, Explanatory Diagrams, Charts and Forms
*   Price/$69.95*

HOLOGRAPHIC HEALTH -- VOLUME III
Air Element, Holopathic Energy Signatures

This is the third of four volumes. It encompasses the element of air. It includes color charts, graphs, and pictures that explain methods of ascertaining information about individual energy imbalances. It contains over 6,500 energy signatures. Everything in existence has its own energy signature. By knowing the correct energy signature, the practitioner is able to re-establish balance within the individual. Volume III is essentially an instruction and reference manual that details some of the most powerful, correlated information on energy re-balancing currently known. This gives the practitioner and layperson a solid foundation upon which to help others who are suffering. As a result, we can find practical solutions for realizing a state of balanced health.

Recommended for Licensed Professionals:
338 pages, ISBN: 0-9619595-7-6
Explanatory Photos and Charts   Price: $49.95

HOLOGRAPHIC HEALTH -- VOLUME IV
Water Element, Holopuncture

Volume IV introduces the study of Holopuncture and its vast applications to modern day health imbalances. It is the final integrated component within the theory and is governed by the element of water. Holopuncture utilizes the Twelve Superstring Pathways which loop and traverse the body, forming a system of 816 holopoints that provide access to the body's twelve holographic systems. Included in this volume are 160 photographs with 55 diagrams, charts and descriptions which allow one to locate the positions of each of the 816 holopoints. Rebalancing modalities and methods are explained and demonstrated.

Holopuncture can be practiced separately with excellent results or can be used in conjunction with knowledge from the other three volumes. This synthesis of information will hasten a truly complete bioenergetic body rebalancing. Practitioners and lay-people alike can learn and benefit. The premise of Holographic Health is to synchronize all aspects of the physical, emotional, mental, and intuitive self with our immortal SOUL.

Recommended for Licensed Professionals:
354 pages, ISBN: 0-9619595-8-4 Price: $59.95

EARTH SAFE
Variable Earth Frequency Harmonizer

Much of the world today is so polluted by harsh and dangerous electromagnetic frequencies that air and water pollution are small problems in comparison. Electricity is just a carrier wave. What comes to your home via your electric company are the aberrant frequencies of your community and the world. The earth frequency was originally found to be 7.83 hertz in 1983, but no longer. It is known that the earth is demagnetizing at a rate of .05% a year. This creates a tremendous stress on all the elements of the earth in every country and ocean.

The result is that the hertz frequency is changing. Over the past 500 years the earth's magnetic field strength has decreased a total of 50%! Your body's biomagnetic field is affected adversely because of this subtle, yet insidious daily hertz frequency change. The effect is now so bad on people's health that there is a syndrome named after it called, "Magnetic Field Deficiency Syndrome".

EARTH SAFE 1, Individual Pocket-sized Harmonizer
(9 volt battery included) Wt. 5 oz. Price: $149.95

EARTH SAFE 2, Whole House Harmonizer
(Uses standard electrical outlet) Wt. 18 oz   Price: $249.95

EARTH SAFE 3, House Harmonizer plus Color Energy Re-Balancer
(Uses standard electrical outlet) Wt. 18 oz   Price: $349.95

OPTIONAL CAR ADAPTER
(for Earth 2 or Earth 3 Only)   Price: $ 9.95

NOTE: The information in this catalog is only for educational purposes. Dr. Baroody does not prescribe, treat, diagnose, or recommend for any health condition and assumes no responsibility. In no way should this information be considered a substitute for competent health care.

To request catalog containing further information and ingredients, please call 1-800-566-1522.

BIOKINETIC FOMULAS

ALKALINE-FORMING SUPPLEMENTS
ORDER FORMS
1-800-566-1522

Product	Amount	Price	Qty	Total
12 Systems Synergistic Multiple Vitamin	100 Tabs	$19.95		
Absolutely Pure L-Glutamine	100 g.	19.95		
Absolutely Pure L-Glutamine	250 g.	39.95		
Alka-Trace	1.25 oz.	5.95		
Alka-Trace *(refill)*	4 oz.	19.95		
Alka-Trace *(refill)*	8 oz.	29.95		
Alpha-Omega	100 Gels	26.95		
Amish Healing Wonder Oil	4 oz.	7.95		
Aneem-Away	8 oz.	9.95		
Aspara-Can	100 Caps	13.95		
At-Eez	100 Tabs	18.95		
Baby Flush *(for sinuses)*	1.25 oz.	1.95		
Back-Off	100 Tabs	17.95		
Bee Powerful	90 Caps	27.95		
Bee the Best	4 oz.	7.95		
B-Well	8 oz.	9.95		
Blood Harmonizer	100 Tabs	19.95		
Calcium Penetrator	100 Tabs	16.95		
Campho-Heal	2 oz.	6.95		
Can-Clear	100 Tabs	18.95		
Cherry Gold	100 Caps	19.95		
Colon-ize	100 Caps	21.95		
Complete-C	100 Tabs	17.95		
Delete	1 oz.	14.95		
Disinfect *(for ears)*	½ oz.	6.95		
Energy-Up	100 Tabs	16.95		
Extreme Greens	100 Caps	19.95		
Eye-C	½ oz.	6.95		
Feel Good	100 Tabs	14.95		
Flow-Thru	100 Tabs	16.95		
Flush Out *(for sinuses)*	2 oz.	7.95		
Free Breath	100 Tabs	17.95		
Fresh Start	2 oz.	11.95		
Fungal Foe	100 Tabs	19.95		
Glyco-Well	90 Caps	21.95		
Great Gums *(for gums)*	2 oz.	10.95		
Heart-Line	100 Tabs	18.95		
Hemorr-mend	1.25 oz.	4.95		
HHS Formula	100 Caps	14.95		
HHS Stomach Egg w/instructions		9.95		

Product	Amount	Price	Qty	Total
Holopathics	180 Pellets	5.95		
Infect Away	100 Caps	16.95		
In-Sync	100 Tabs	18.95		
Kleen Sweep	100 Caps	17.95		
Magnesium Penetrator	100 Tabs	17.95		
Magnets: 4000 gauss	Each	1.95		
Minotaur *(4 sizes, call for pricing)*	100 g.	12.95		
Myo-Majestic *(4 sizes, call for pricing)*	100 g.	16.95		
Myo-My! *(4 sizes, call for pricing)*	100 g.	18.95		
Mood Mender	100 Tabs	19.95		
Nail-Well	0.5 oz.	11.95		
Ouch-Away	2 oz.	14.95		
Pink Lady *(crème)*	1.25 oz.	9.95		
Pan-Gest	100 Tabs	21.95		
Para-Go-Way	240 Tabs	17.95		
Protector	100 Tabs	19.95		
Pro-Tone *(crème)*	0.75 oz.	11.95		
Racket Free	2 oz.	19.95		
Senses	100 Tabs	17.95		
Sungold *(crème)*	1.25 oz.	11.95		
Symmetry	100 Tabs	19.95		
The Recipe	4 oz.	7.95		
Tri-Force	100 Tabs	17.95		
Trim-Silver *(nighttime)*	60 Tabs	21.95		
Weight Loss System- A Balanced Approach	3 Items	54.95		
Wipe-Out	100 g.	19.95		
Wipe-Out	250 g.	39.95		
Women's Booster	100 Tabs	17.95		
Zinc Penetrator	100 Tabs	18.95		
Books/Media				
Alkalize or Die		14.95		
Alkalize or Die Book and Chart Combo		24.95		
Ascension: Beginner's Manual 1		12.95		
Ascension: Beginner's Manual 2		17.95		
Asparagus Can Do it For You		4.95		
Brotherhood of Intuition		3.95		
Hiatal Hernia Syndrome		13.95		
Hiatal Hernia Book, Formula, and Egg Combo		29.95		
Holographic Health Volume I (Earth)		39.95		
Holographic Health Volume II (Fire)		69.95		
Holographic Health Volume III (Air)		49.95		
Holographic Health Volume IV (Water)		59.95		
80%/20% -- Alkaline-Acid Chart		14.95		
Earth Safe I, Personal Size Unit		149.95		

Product	Amount	Price	Qty	Total
Earth Safe II, Whole House Unit		249.95		
Earth Safe III, Whole House w/color balancer		349.95		
Alkaline/Acid Water Test Kit		17.95		
Sub-total For First Page				
Sub-total For Second Page				
Sub-total For Third Page				
Total				

MAIL TO:
HOLOGRAPHIC HEALTH®, INC
119 Pigeon St., Waynesville, NC 28786
Call: 1-800-566-1522 / Fax: 1-828-456-8787 /
E-Mail: *Holographichlth@aol.com* / Website: *WWW.Holographichealth.com*

Subotal	
Sales Tax *(NC Residents Only)* 7.0%	
Shipping Charge(UPS: $7.00 for the 1st lb. & $0.50 for each additional lb.)	
Total Due	

Phone # You Can Be Reached At: *Failure To Provide # May Delay Your Order*
Home Phone: **Cell Phone:**

Bill To:
Name:
Billing Address:
Street:

City: State: Zip

Ship To:
Name:
Ship To Address (No PO Box Numbers For UPS Delivery):
Street:

City: State: Zip

Credit Card # **Expiration Date**
   -      -   - Exp:

Mastercard	Visa	Discover	Check Money Order
☐	☐	☐	☐

Signature

Make Checks Payable To: Holographic Health®, Inc.

Revised 1/2007